Hormonal Actions in Non-endocrine Systems

Hormonal Actions
in Non-endocrine
Systems

Edited by
Walter B. Essman
Departments of Psychology and Biochemistry
Queens College of the City University of New York
Flushing, New York

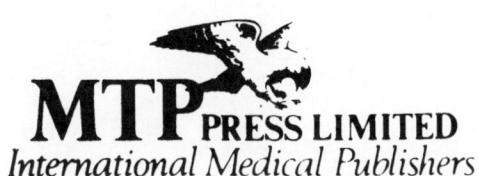
MTP **PRESS LIMITED**
International Medical Publishers

Published in the UK and Europe by
MTP Press Limited
Falcon House
Lancaster, England

Published in the US by
SPECTRUM PUBLICATIONS, INC.
175-20 Wexford Terrace
Jamaica, NY 11432

ISBN-13: 978-94-009-6603-1   e-ISBN-13: 978-94-009-6601-7
DOI: 10.1007/978-94-009-6601-7

Preface

The actions of hormones upon systems outside of the usual target sites for such molecules represents an area of increasing interest and growing clinical significance. This volume represents a cross-section of such actions of hormones upon several relevant sites.

In the first chapter of this volume Dr. Malick discusses the current status of endorphins as analgesic agents. It is now known that a more primary level of control exists for β-endorphin in that a 41-amino acid peptide has been isolated from ovine hypothalamus; this peptide stimulates β-endorphin release as well as the secretion of corticotropin (Vale et al., 1981). The analgesic properties of corticotropin and its immunoactive-like analogs are well known, so it does not come as a surprise that these two classes of analgesic peptides are regulated by a common hypothalamic control peptide. It may also be of interest to observe that an increase in β-endorphin concentration in the pituitary occurs in genetically obese mice and rats, and that such obesity can be attenuated through the administration of nalaxone (Margules et al., 1978). It has also been determined that genetically obese mice have a probable cholecystokinin deficiency in the cerebral cortex in that this peptide is a satiety-inducing agent (Saito, et al., 1981). The analgesic properties of the latter have also been observed.

The extra-pituitary actions of another pituitary peptide, as examined in the second chapter of this volume by Dr. Hirsch, while indicating the nature of TRH receptors in several brain regions and how these interact with barbiturates, concerns essentially sites, although outside of the pituitary, still within the brain. The feedback of peripheral hormone status upon the pituitary can in turn affect the pituitary response to TRH. A case in point is that males with primary testicular failure show an exaggerated response of prolactin release to the administration of TRH (Spitz et al., 1980), an effect that may be mediated by estrogen. The predictable release of prolactin by TRH under normal circumstances may play a role in the regulatory effects of TRH outside of the pituitary. In addition, it may be observed that specific membrane receptor sites for TRH have been identified in fetal sheep thyroid cells (Essman et al., 1980), which could well represent only one of several non-brain extra pituitary sites upon which TRH is capable of exerting a regulatory function.

Some of the functions of the gastrointestinal hormones were explored by Dr. Misra in a previous volume (1980) and in the present book he and Dr. Baruh consider some of the diagnostic and therapeutic roles of these agents. In this regard some attention may be called to a familial glucogonoma syndrome (Stacpoole et al., 1981) in which a pancreatic A cell neoplasm was documented in family members. There may also be note taken that there are a reasonably large number of nonfunctioning islet cell tumors in which there is no clinical evidence of hormone production. It may also be observed that hormones acting upon the gastrointestinal tract and secondarily upon G.I. hormones, can alter the gastric mucosa; glucagon is capable of protecting the gastric mucosa against aspirin-induced injury (Stachura et al., 1981) and adaptive mucosal hyperplasia has been observed from elevated levels of enteroglucagon. The changes in gastric and colonic smooth muscle in response to proinsulin, insulin, and motilin are well known, but the effects of the latter upon gastric emptying appear to be specific for glucose rather than fats (Chistofedes et al., 1981). There is a possibility that gastric fat content may serve to interfere with the gastric mucosal effects of motilin.

In Chapter 4 the issue of perinatal hypothyroidism and brain function is considered. It might be appropriate to consider that a resistance to thyroid hormone could serve independently as a basis for CNS effects, especially since a familial entity of this type has been reported (Bartato et al., 1981). An altered response of the pituitary to thyroxine or to TRH could account for a receptor-mediated hormonal failure, which if present during perinatal development could profoundly influence brain function.

The actions of thyroid hormones on the lung, as explored in Chapter 5 by Drs. Das and Steinberg, concerns a highly original relationship that has suggested important regulatory functions for thyroid hormones in pulmonary status. Changes in thyroid status, the dependence of phospholipid synthesis in the lung upon thyroid hormones and the requirement of specific phospholipids at those sites in the lung to which thyroid hormones bind suggest that specific lung cells may contain sites that autoregulate in response to the availability of thyroid hormones. This holds potential clinical significance, not only for the lung as a target site that may be affected in thyroid dysfunction, but also that alterations in pulmonary function may modify the response of specific lung sites to thyroid hormones during critical periods of growth and development. The issue also brings into play a possible therapeutic role for thyroid hormones in pulmonary disorders, such that altered lung mechanics, gas exchange, or drug absorption may be modified.

In the final chapter of this volume, Drs. Chitkara and Khan have undertaken the ambitious task of discussing the hormonal status of the lung and also have pointed to some of the functions that these endogenous principles underlie. A very important role for some of the endogenous hormones of the lung is as markers for carcinomas of the lung. Recent important observations (Berger et al., 1981), measurement of L-dopa-decarboxylase, histaminase, calcitonin, and β-endorphin in samples of pulmonary neoplasms indicated a wide range of variability for different tumor types with only minimal selectivity shown; for example, adenocarcinomas or large cell carcinomas did not contain β-endorphin, whereas very high calcitonin levels were found in the former. At least two, or more markers were associated with small cell carcinomas. Whether hormone marker profiles will characterize the type of lung carcinoma or predict size, extent of metastases, or response to therapy remains to be studied, however, there can be little doubt that the lung is a significant site for hormone production.

The present volume is the result only of the cooperation and patience of its contributors, who took time from busy clinical and research activities to provide a current and usable guide to those subjects in which they are experts. Such expertise from fields as pharmacology, psychology, gastroenterology, metabolism, biochemistry, and pulmonary medicine, made my job, as editor, a most enjoyable one. It is my hope that the reader will find, as I did, that there is much to be learned about the influences of hormones upon most endocrine sites.

WALTER B. ESSMAN

Flushing, N.Y.
May, 1983

Contents

Contributors

Selim Baruh, M.D.
Division of Diabetes and Metabolism
Department of Medicine
Queens Hospital Center
Jamaica, N.Y.

Rajinder K. Chitkara, M.D.
Division of Pulmonary Medicine
Department of Medicine
Queens Hospital Center
Jamaica, N.Y.

Dipak K. Das, Ph.D.
Division of Pulmonary Medicine
Department of Medicine
Long Island Jewish-Hillside Medical
  Center
New Hyde Park, N.Y.

Walter B. Essman, M.D., Ph.D.
Departments of Psychology
  and Biochemistry
Queens College, of the City
  University of New York
Flushing, N.Y.

Michael D. Hirsch, Ph.D.
Roche Institute for Molecular
  Biology
Nutley, New Jersey

Faroque A. Khan, M.D.
Division of Pulmonary Medicine
Department of Medicine
Queens Hospital Center
Jamaica, N.Y.

Jeffrey B. Malick, Ph.D.
Division of Neuropharmacology
I.C.I.
Wilmington, Delaware

Prem Misra, M.D.
Division of Gastroenterology
Department of Medicine
Queens Hospital Center
Jamaica, N.Y.

Harry Steinberg, M.D.
Division of Pulmonary Medicine
Department of Medicine
Long Island Jewish-Hillside Medical
  Center
New Hyde Park, N.Y.

1

Analgesic Activity of Endorphins

JEFFREY B. MALICK

The demonstration that electrical stimulation of the mesencephalic gray in rats produced a profound analgesic response was one of the earliest reports providing experimental evidence suggestive of the presence of endogenous morphine-like substances in the brain (Reynolds, 1969). The analgesia produced by the electrical brain stimulation was sufficient to permit a laparotomy to be performed (Reynolds, 1969). Subsequent reports have demonstrated that electrical stimulation of medial brain stem regions, especially the periaqueductal gray (PAG), resulted in potent analgesic activity in the rat (Balagura and Ralph, 1973; Mayer and Libeskind, 1974), cat (Liebeskind et al., 1973; Oliveras et al., 1974), rhesus monkey (Goodman and Holcombe, 1976) and man (Adams, 1976; Richardson and Akil, 1973); Mayer and Price (1976) have written an excellent review on brain stimulation-induced analgesia.

Brain stimulation-induced analgesia is significantly antagonized by naloxone, a narcotic antagonist (Adams, 1976; Akil et al., 1976). In addition, microinjection of morphine into the PAG resulted in marked naloxone-reversible analgesic activity (Herz et al., 1970; Pert and Yaksh, 1974) and brain stimulation-induced analgesia exhibited both tolerance (Mayer and Hayes, 1975) and cross-tolerance to morphine administered at the same brain site (Mayer and Hayes, 1975; Mayer and Murphin, 1976). Therefore, it was believed that the electrical stimulation caused the release of some endogenous substance that resulted in an opiate-like analgesic response.

Goldstein and associates (1971) discovered a method for detecting the presence of opiate receptors in mouse brain. This discovery generated a flurry of research activity in this area and, as a result, within two years several laboratories had independently demonstrated the occurrence of stereospecific opiate receptor binding sites in brain (Pert and Snyder, 1973; Simon et al., 1973; Terenius, 1973). Obviously, these opiate binding sites were not present in brain merely to accommodate the poppy alkaloids; therefore, several laboratories throughout the world intensified their search for the endogenous morphine-like substances.

Hughes and associates (1975) discovered two pentapeptides in extracts of porcine brain that produced morphinomimetic activity when tested on their guinea pig ileum and mouse vas deferens preparations. They named these peptides methionine-enkephalin and leucine-enkephalin, and noted that the methionine form was approximately four times as prevalent in whole pig brain as the leucine form (Hughes et al., 1975). These pentapeptides only differed from one another structurally in their terminal amino acid and they were identified as Tyr-Gly-Gly-Phe-Met and Tyr-Gly-Gly-Phe-Leu, met-enkephalin and leu-enkephalin, respectively. In their original paper (Hughes et al., 1975) the authors pointed out the interesting and important observation that the sequence of met-enkephalin was present in the structure of β-lipotropin (β-LPH residues 61-65) (see Figure 1); this peptide hormone containing 91 amino acids had been isolated from pituitary glands as early as 1964. Three additional segments of β-LPH with opiate-like activity were isolated from brain and pituitary extracts (Bradbury et al., 1976; Cox et al., 1976; Lazarus et al., 1976; Ling et al., 1976; Ling and Guillemin, 1976): β-endorphin (β-LPH 61-76); γ-endorphin (β-LPH 61-77), and β-endorphin (β-LPH 61-91; C-fragment) (see Figure 1).

H-Glu . . . . . Tyr-Gly-Gly-Phe-Met-Thr-Ser-
　　1　　　　　61　　　　　　　65

Glu-Lys-Ser-Gln-Thr-Pro-Leu-Val-Thr-
　　　　　　　　　　　　　76

Leu-Phe-Lys-Asn-Ala-Ile-Ile Lys-Asn-
77

Ala-Tyr-Lys-Lys-Gly-Glu-OH
　　　　　91

Fig. 1. The amino acid sequence of various endorphins in human β-lipotropin: met-enkephalin (β-LPH 61-65); α-endorphin (β-LPH 61-76); γ-endorphin (β-LPH 61-77); β-endorphin (β-LPH 61-91).

As in any area in which the research and discoveries proceed very rapidly, the nomenclature does not always evolve in a systematic manner. Hughes and co-workers (1975) named their peptides enkephalins. However, Eric Simon coined the term endorphins in 1975 and since then this has been used as a generic descriptor for the endogenous morphine-like substances.

The purpose of this chapter is to survey the literature on the analgesic activity of the endorphins and to speculate as to their possible relevance in pain mechanisms, especially in terms of pain syndromes observed clinically in humans.

EFFECTS OF ENDORPHINS IN TESTS PREDICTIVE OF ANALGESIC ACTIVITY

This section will summarize the results of the many experiments that have been performed to assess the analgesic potential of the naturally occurring opiate-like substances (endorphins); the intent is to discuss the endogenous compounds and to omit any discussion of the many synthetic endorphins, several of which appear to be extremely potent antinociceptive agents in animals.

The bulk of the discussion will deal with the activities of methionine-enkephalin, leucine-enkephalin, and β-endorphin. However, brief mention will be made of the activity of β-lipotropin and several of the other endorphins (e.g., α-endorphin, γ-endorphin) that have been discovered in animals and humans and that could have a physiologic role in the organism.

Methionine-Enkephalin

Table 1 summarizes the results of the analgesic studies performed on methionine-enkephalin in various laboratories. In April 1976 Belluzzi and co-workers (1976) were the first to report analgesic activity following the central administration of enkephalins to rats. In this study rats were implanted stereotaxically with permanently indwelling cannulae, the tips of which were located in the lateral ventricle. One week after surgery the rats were tested in the tail flick test (D'Amour and Smith, 1941) for analgesic activity following the intracerebroventricular infusion of methionine-enkephalin. The tail flick test has been used frequently to evaluate the analgesic potential of the endorphins since it readily detects opiate drugs (e.g., morphine) (Bloom et al., 1976). Follow-

Table 1. Effects of Methionine-Enkephalin in Various Analgesic Tests in Rodents and Cats.

Investigator(s)	Species	Analgesic Model	Route of Administration	Dose (μg)	Injection Volume (μl)	Analgesic Activity
Belluzzi et al. (1976)	Rat	Tail flick	i.c.v.[a]	100, 200	10	Significant analgesia at both doses; onset (2-6 minutes); duration (10-12 minutes)
Büscher et al. (1976)	Mouse	Tail flick	i.v.[b]	Several[c]	—[d]	ED_{50} = 170 mg/kg; 15-second duration
	Mouse	Tail flick	i.c.v.	56-180	10-30	ED_{50} = 75 (52-100); peak activity (2 minutes); duration (5 minutes)
Chang et al. (1976)	Rat	Tail flick	i.c. (PAG)[e]	30-360	3	Sign. analgesia only at 120 μg/rat; duration $<$3 minutes
Feldberg and Smyth (1976)	Cat	Tail pinch	i.c.v.	50-400	40	No analgesic activity
	Cat	Tail pinch	i.v.	1 mg/kg	—[d]	No analgesic activity
Graf et al. (1976)	Rat	Tail flick	i.c.v.	670 nmoles	20	Slight analgesia; duration (8 minutes)

Table 1 (Continued)

Reference	Species	Test	Route			Result
Leybin et al. (1976)	Rat	Hot plate (44.5°C)	i.c.v.	100	10	No analgesia; apparent increase in pain perception (increased paw licking)
Loh et al. (1976)	Mouse	Tail flick / Hot plate / Acetic acid writhing	i.c.v.	50	5	Weak analgesic activity; duration <10 minutes
Malick and Goldstein (1976, 1977)	Rat	Tail flick	i.c. (PAG)	4.8–48	1	ED_{50} = 15.5 (9.9–24.2) μg/rat; peak activity (1 minute); short duration (dropping off by 7 minutes)
Ronai et al. (1976)	Rat	Tail flick	i.c.v.	400	20	Moderate prolongation of reaction times; duration: 4–6 minutes
Bradbury et al. (1977)	Rat	Hot plate (55.5°C)	i.c.v.	100	10	Transient analgesia; 10-minute duration; N = 1
Meglio et al. (1977)	Cat	Tooth pulp	i.c.v.	100–400	500	No analgesic activity
	Cat	Pinch test (tail, limbs, ears)	i.c.v.	100–400	500	No analgesic activity

Table 1 (Continued)

Investigator(s)	Species	Analgesic Model	Route of Administration	Dose (μg)	Injection Volume (μl)	Analgesic Activity
Roemer et al. (1977)	Mouse	Tail flick	i.c.v.	Several[c]	—[d]	ED_{50} = 68 μg/mouse at 2 minute postinfusion
Szekely et al. (1977a)	Rat	Tail flick	i.c.v.	Several[c]	20	Weak analgesic activity; impossible to calculate an ED_{50} as high as 6.7×10^{-7} mole/rat
Urca et al. (1977)	Rat	Tail flick	i.c.v.	200	10	8/13 drug naive rats exhibited significant analgesia; duration 1–40 minutes (median = 4 minutes)
Walker et al. (1977)	Rat	Tail flick	i.c.v.	200	10	Slight, significant analgesia; maximum increase in latency = 2.0 seconds; duration = 4 minutes

[a]Intracerebroventricular
[b]Intravenous
[c]Actual doses not reported
[d]Not reported
[e]Intracerebral; periaqueductal gray

ing the administration of methionine-enkephalin (100 and 200 μg/ rat, i.c.v.), statistically significant, dose-related increases in tail flick response) were observed. The analgesia produced by the highest dose (200 μg/rat) of methionine-enkephalin appeared to be equivalent to that produced by a 10-μg/rat dose of morphine sulfate; thus, although methionine-enkephalin produced significant analgesia, it was approximately 20 times less potent than morphine when administered into the ventricles.

Methionine-enkephalin exhibited a rapid onset (2–6 minutes) of analgesic activity, which also rapidly disappeared by 10–12 minutes postdrug infusion. The delay between the time of administration and the onset of activity was most likely attributable to diffusion time to the active sites and the short duration of activity was probably due to the rapid catabolism of enkephalins by brain enzymes (Hughes, 1975). Since pretreatment with naloxone (2 mg/kg, s.c.), a pure narcotic antagonist, significantly antagonized the analgesic activity produced by methionine-enkephalin, it appeared to produce this activity by an interaction with opiate receptors.

At approximately the same time (April 1976) that the first publication in this area (Belluzzi et al., 1976) appeared, an abstract was submitted by Malick and Goldstein (1976) for presentation at the Fall Pharmacology Meeting (New Orleans, La., August 1976); the expanded manuscript appeared in early 1977 (Malick and Goldstein, 1977). This study was the first in which complete dose-response curves were generated in order to compare the analgesic potencies of methionine-enkephalin and morphine via the potency ratio analysis of Litchfield and Wilcoxon (1949). In this study rats were stereotaxically implanted with cannulae located in the dorsal border of the raphe nucleus in the midbrain periaqueductal gray (PAG). This site was chosen because it had been shown to be one of the primary sites in the brain at which morphine exhibits potent analgesic activity. The methodology used in this study is discussed briefly as an example of the procedures commonly utilized in many of the studies reported here.

In studies in which drugs are to be infused directly into the brain, rats are generally allowed at least a week to recover fully from the trauma associated with the surgical implantation of the guide cannula. All rats are then tested for their responsiveness to the noxious stimulus, which in the case of the tail flick procedure is radiant heat, following the infusion of the vehicle (sterile water in this study) in which the test drugs have been dissolved; such studies are used as control baselines and are absolutely necessary to assure that the rat does not respond to the vehicle alone. Any animal that exhibited a significant alteration from control baselines following control (vehicle) infusion would have been eliminated from the study; in the study being discussed, none of the subjects exhibited a significant change following vehicle infusion. Infusions are accomplished by inserting an internal cannula into the permanently implanted guide cannula; the internal cannula extends 2 mm beyond the tip of the guide cannula. An infusion pump is used to deliver a small volume (1 μl or less into tissue) relatively slowly and at a constant rate; in the present study drugs were infused in a 1 μl volume over 24 seconds (infusion rate = 0.04 μl/second). The internal cannula should be left in place for a short period of time (e.g., 25 seconds) to prevent the infused fluid from immediately flowing back up the guide cannula. Rats were then placed in a standard Plexiglas restrainer so that only the tail protruded. Control sessions were performed on the morning of each day of drug testing and consisted of infusion of sterile water and testing for tail flick responses (latency to respond) at 1, 3, and 7 minutes postinfusion. After establishing same-day control thresholds for each rat, drugs were infused and tail flick latencies were measured once again at the same intervals postinfusion. Thus each rat served as its own control. Any rat exhibiting a 50% or greater increase in response latency as compared with the rat's own same-day control value was considered to have shown a significant analgesic response. If the rat did not respond within 20 seconds, the heat source was terminated in order to prevent tissue damage. When animals were used more than once, at least seven days were allowed between drug administrations in an attempt to avoid the development of tolerance. The results of this study are summarized in Table 2.

When infused directly into the PAG, both morphine and methionine-enkephalin exhibited potent, dose-related analgesic activity (Table 2). Methionine-enkephalin was approximately four times less potent than morphine on a weight basis; however, if the potency comparison were based on the molar ED_{50} ratio, the potency of met-enkephalin would be increased by a factor of 2 relative to morphine (i.e., molar ED_{50} s: met-enkephalin = 0.27 μmoles; morphine = 0.13 μmoles). Thus met-enkephalin was found to be much more potent in the study by Malick and Goldstein (1977) as compared with the results obtained by Belluzzi et al. (1976). This difference in potency most likely arises from the fact that Belluzzi and his associates utilized the intraventricular route of administration, which required diffusion to the site(s) of action. This could have dramatically reduced the activity of the peptide as enkephalins have been shown to be rapidly deactivated

Table 2. Analgesic Activity of Methionine-Enkephalin and Morphine in the Tail Flick Test in Rats Following Intracerebral Administration[a]

Treatment	Dose ($\mu g/rat$)	N[b]	% Rats Exhibiting a Significant Increase in Response Latency[c]	ED_{50} ($\mu g/rat$) (95% CL)[d]
Sterile water	1 μl	133	0.0	—
Morphine SO_4 (7 minutes)[e]	1.7	7	28.6	3.7
	3.0	7	28.6	(2.2–6.1)
	10.0	10	80.0	
		9	100.0	
Met-enkephalin (1 minute)[e]	4.8	19	21.1	15.5
	9.6	17	35.3	(9.9–24.2)
	16.0	19	47.4	
	48.0	16	81.3	

[a]Data from Malick and Goldstein (1977)
[b]Number of rats tested
[c]Any rat exhibiting a 50% or greater increase in response latency was considered to be significantly affected
[d]ED_{50} and 95% confidence limits were calculated by the method of Litchfield and Wilcoxon (1949)
[e]Data from time of peak activity

by peptidases in brain and other tissue (Hambrook et al., 1976). Following intracerebral infusion (PAG), the analgesic activity of met-enkephalin peaked by 1 minute postinfusion but had a very short duration of activity (its activity had significantly diminished by 7 minutes postinfusion); this is in agreement with the short duration of activity reported by Belluzzi and co-workers (1976). In contrast, the activity of morphine did not peak until the 7-minute observation time but persisted for as long as several hours postinfusion, which is consistent with previous observations (Yaksh et al., 1976). The analgesic activity of met-enkephalin was completely antagonized by pretreatment with the narcotic receptor antagonist, naloxone (see Table 3). The high dose of naloxone (20 mg/kg, i.p.) used in this antagonism study was chosen since previous studies had demonstrated that although much lower doses will antagonize parenteral doses of morphine, relatively high doses of the antagonist are necessary to antagonize morphine-induced analgesia following direct infusion into the periaqueductal gray.

In contrast to the studies of Malick and Goldstein (1977), Chang et al. (1976) reported that methionine-enkephalin was at least 20 times less potent than morphine in the tail flick test in

Table 3.   Inhibition of Analgesic Activity by Pretreatment with Naloxone

Treatment	Dose (μg/rat)	Number of Rats Significantly Affected[a]/Number of Rats Tested (Mean % Change in Response Latency[b])		P-Value[d]
		Drug Alone	Drug + Naloxone[c]	
Sterile water	1 μl	0/28 (—)	0/28 (—)	—
Morphine SO$_4$	10	9/9 (201.55)	3/9 (30.84)	<0.001
Met-enkephalin	48	10/10 (168.01)	0/10 (5.59)	<0.001

[a]Data from time of peak activity
[b]Mean percent change in response latency =

$$\frac{\text{Mean predrug threshold} - \text{Mean postdrug threshold}}{\text{Mean predrug threshold}} \times 100$$

[c]Naloxone HCl (20 mg/kg, i.p.) 30 minutes prior to drug infusion
[d]Paired Student's t-test comparing mean percent change in response latency for drug + naloxone with drug alone

rats following infusion into the PAG; however, in their study no dose–response relationship was observed (significant activity was exhibited at 120 μg/rat but not at 30 or 360 μg/rat). Met-enkephalin was also shown to be markedly less potent than morphine following intraventricular administration in mice when tested in the tail flick procedure (Büscher et al., 1976). Although morphine was found to be 75 times more potent than met-enkephalin, the potency ratio could have been biased once again in favor of morphine because of the route of administration, which would make compounds that were rapidly degraded appear less potent than those that are not when administered at locations that were not the sites of such activity. Büscher and co-workers also reported analgesic activity in the mouse tail flock model following intravenous administration (ED$_{50}$ = 170 mg/kg, i.v.); however, the analgesic activity only lasted for 15 seconds.

Several other laboratories have also shown that met-enkephalin produces significant, although frequently weak, analgesic activity in the tail flick test following intraventricular administration in both rats (Graf et al., 1976; Ronai et al., 1976; Szekely et al., 1977a; Urca et al., 1977; Walker et al., 1977) and mice (Loh et al., 1976; Roemer et al., 1977). (See Table 1 for details).

Another analgesia model in rodents that has been routinely used to evaluate opiate analgesics is the hot plate procedure in rats and mice (Eddy and Leimbach, 1953; Fraser and Harris, 1967; Cochin, 1968; Dewey and Harris, 1971). In the original version of the hot plate procedure the temperature of the surface of the plate was maintained at 54–56°C by the vapors of a boiling solvent, usually pure acetone or a mixture of solvents (Cochin, 1968; Johannesson and Woods, 1964). However, with the advent of modern technology, it is now possible electronically to maintain the platform surface very accurately at any desired temperature (Goldstein and Malick, 1979). Briefly, rodents are placed on the surface of the test platform within the confines of a bell jar or other container and are observed for reactions to the heat-induced pain. The end points vary from laboratory to laboratory but usually consist of licking of the paws, the rapid lifting of a paw, or an attempt to escape from the area. A cut-off time (standardly 30 or 60 seconds) is used to prevent tissue damage, which is especially critical if the animals are to be tested more than once.

Utilizing the hot plate procedure, Bradbury and associates (1977) demonstrated a transient analgesic response (approximately 10 minutes in duration) following a total dose of 100 μg intraventricularly in the only rat tested. However, Leybin and co-workers (1976) administered an identical dose (100 μg/rat, i.c.v.) and failed to observe any analgesic response; in fact, they apparently observed hyperalgesia (an increase in paw licking). Surprisingly, they reported that the animals that received met-enkephalin exhibited signs of narcotic withdrawal (e.g., wet dog shakes, restlessness, stereotypy, defecation) 1–3 minutes after the initiation of drug infusion. The differences in these results cannot be easily reconciled; whereas no analgesia was observed at 45.5°C, a significant response was observed at the higher temperature, 55.5°C (Bradbury et al., 1977). In mice intraventricular administration of met-enkephalin (50 μg/mouse) resulted in significant analgesia that lasted for less than 10 minutes (Loh et al., 1976).

Chemically induced writhing (abdominal constriction) models in mice have been used frequently to assess analgesic potential. These models detect analgesic activity with both narcotic and nonnarcotic analgesics (Brittain et al., 1963; Chernov et al., 1967; Taber et al., 1969). Loh and co-workers (1976) demonstrated weak antinociceptive activity following met-enkephalin (50 μg/ mouse, i.c.v.) in the acetic acid-induced writhing test (Table 1).

In cats, Feldberg and Smyth (1976) failed to demonstrate analgesia with met-enkephalin in the tail pinch test following either intraventricular (50–400 μg) or intravenous (1 mg/kg) administration. Meglio et al. (1977) also failed to observe analgesic activity in cats in utilizing pinch procedures (pinching tail, limbs, or ears) following intraventricular administration of met-enkephalin over a wide range of doses (100–400 μg/cat, i.c.v.). In the electrically stimulated tooth pulp model, met-enkephalin was also found to be ineffective in cats (100–400 μg/cat, i.c.v.).

Thus met-enkephalin has not been shown to be an analgesic in the cat to date, utilizing tooth pulp or pinch procedures. This may be due either to species differences or to the different types of analgesic methodologies that have been used in cats thus far, none of which have been utilized to assess the analgesic potential of met-enkephalin in rodents.

In summary, met-enkephalin has been shown to produce significant analgesic activity in rodents in several different types of analgesic procedures (i.e., hot plate, tail flick, writhing) following intraventricular administration. If the drug was infused (i.c.) directly into the site at which morphine is active (e.g., PAG), then activity almost comparable to that observed with morphine was observed (Malick and Goldstein, 1976, 1977). However, if met-enkephalin was placed into the ventricles where it had to diffuse to the site of action, it appeared to be much less potent than morphine, but this is probably due to rapid catabolism prior to the peptide reaching its receptor site. In one study (Büscher et al., 1976) met-enkephalin exhibited weak activity in the mouse tail flick procedure following intravenous administration.

Leucine-Enkephalin

Whereas met-enkephalin has been investigated extensively for its analgesic potential, only a handful of investigators have evaluated leu-enkaphalin as an analgesic. The results of these studies are summarized in Table 4.

As with met-enkephalin, Belluzzi and co-workers (1976) were the first to report that leu-enkephalin produces a statistically significant analgesic response when infused directly into the brain of rats (see Table 4). Following intraventricular administration of leu-enkephalin (100 and 200 μg/rat, i.c.v.), a significant prolongation of tail flick latencies was observed. The onset of this activity occurred at 2 to 6 minutes postdrug infusion and the duration of the analgesic activity was very short (10–12 minutes). In this study intraventricular administration of a dose of 10 μg of morphine produced an equivalent analgesic response to that observed after the highest dose (200 μg/rat) of leu-enkephalin tested; the duration of morphine's activity was also considerably longer ($>$1 hour) than that observed with leu-enkephalin. The analgesic response of leu-enkephalin was also reversed by treatment with a narcotic antagonist, naloxone (2 mg/kg, s.c.) (Belluzzi et al., 1976).

Table 4. Effects of Leucine-Enkephalin in Analgesic Tests in Rodents

Investigator(s)	Species	Analgesic Model	Route of Administration	Dose (μg)	Injection Volume (μl)	Analgesic Activity
Belluzzi et al. (1976)	Rat	Tail flick	i.c.v.[a]	100,200	10	Significant analgesia at both doses; onset (2-6 minutes); duration: 10-12 minutes
Büscher et al. (1976)	Mouse	Tail flick	i.v.[b]	320 (mg/kg)	–[c]	Weakly active in 4/10 mice
	Mouse	Tail flick	i.c.v.	180-420	10-30	$ED_{50} = 240$ (159-363) μg/mouse; peak activity at 2 minutes; duration = 5 minutes
Chang et al. (1976)	Rat	Tail flick	i.c. (PAG)[d]	30-360	3	No analgesic activity
Leybin et al. (1976)	Rat	Hot plate (44.5°C)	i.c.v.	100	10	Significant analgesia for at least 10 minutes
Malick and Goldstein	Rat	Tail flick	i.c. (PAG)	6-24	1	$ED_{50} = 14.8$ (9.4-23.2) μg/rat; peak activity (3 minutes); activity dropping off by 7 minutes but still significant

[a]Intracerebroventricular
[b]Intravenous
[c]Not reported
[d]Intracerebral; periaqueductal gray

Malick and Goldstein (1976, 1977) also demonstrated, that leu-enkephalin exhibits analgesic activity in a rat tail flick test, however, in their study they admonistered the drugs intracerebrally directly into one of the sites of action of morphine, the PAG. The major reason for infusing the drugs directly into the PAG rather than into the ventricles was to overcome the problems associated with diffusion: for example, because these pentapeptides are rapidly catabolized, most of their activity would be lost before they actually reached the appropriate receptor sites. Malick and Goldstein (1977) were the first to generate a complete dose-response curve and to establish an ED_{50} dose for producing significant analgesia with leu-enkephalin (see Table 5). In their test leu-enkephalin exhibited an ED_{50} of 14.8 µg/rat, i.c., as compared with 3.7 µg/rat for morphine. Reaching peak activity by 3 minutes postinfusion, this activity significantly diminished by 7 minutes postdrug. On a molar basis, leu-enkephalin was only two times less potent than morphine when given in the PAG; that is, molar ED_{50}'s were 0.27 and 0.13 µmoles for leu-enkephalin and morphine respectively. Once again, pretreatment (30 minutes prior to leu-enkephalin) with naloxone (20 mg/kg, i.p.) prevented the analgesic activity of leu-enkephalin (Malick and Goldstein, 1977).

Leybin et al. (1976) reported that leu-enkephalin (100 µg/rat, i.c.v.) produced a significant analgesic response that lasted for at least 10 minutes after infusion into the lateral ventricle when tested in the hot plate test. The temperature of the plate was 44.5°C and the end point used to detect a painful response was hindpaw locking. Naturally, morphine also produced a significant analgesic response in their model. However, interestingly, under the same conditions they failed to demonstrate any analgesic activity with met-enkephalin (100 µg/rat, i.c.v.); in contrast, they found that met-enkephalin produced a hyperalgesic response (i.e., the mean latency to the first hindpaw lick was shorter than when the same animals were infused with physiologic saline).

Büscher and associates (1976) evaluated leu-enkephalin in the tail flick test in mice and found that it exhibited weak but significant analgesic activity (ED_{50} = 240 µg/mouse) following intraventricular administration—an activity that peaked rapidly and disappeared very quickly (see Table 4). In the same studies leu-enkephalin also produced significant but weak analgesia in 40% of the mice tested following intravenous (320 mg/kg) dosing (Table 4). The same studies also showed met-enkephalin to be approximately three times as potent as leu-enkephalin following intraventricular administration. Another interesting observation

Table 5. Comparative Analgesic Activity of Leucine-Enkephalin and Morphine in the Tail Flick Test in Rats Following Intracerebral Administration into the PAG[a]

Treatment	Dose (μg/rat)	N[b]	% Rats Exhibiting a Significant Increase in Response Latency[c]	ED_{50} (μg/rat) (95% CL)[d]
Sterile water	1 μl	133	0.0	—
Leu-enkephalin (3 minutes)[e]	6.0	14	7.1	14.8
	12.0	7	42.9	(9.4–23.2)
	24.0	8	75.0	
Morphine SO_4 (7 minutes)[e]	1.7	7	28.6	3.7
	3.0	7	28.6	(2.2–6.1)
	6.0	10	80.0	
	10.0	9	100.0	

[a] Data from Malick and Goldstein (1977)
[b] Number of rats tested
[c] Any rat exhibiting a 50% or greater increase in response latency was considered to be significantly affected
[d] ED_{50} and 95% confidence limits were calculated by the method of Litchfield and Wilcoxon (1949)
[e] Data from time of peak activity

from these studies was that it required a significantly higher dose of naloxone to antagonize the analgesic response of leu-enkephalin as opposed to the amount necessary to antagonize the effects of either met-enkephalin or morphine. A dose of naloxone as low as 0.1 mg/kg, s.c., could inhibit the analgesic activity of both met-enkephalin or morphine, whereas 10 mg/kg, s.c., was necessary to inhibit the actions of leu-enkephalin. Büscher and co-workers suggested that the different susceptibilities of the two enkephalins to inhibition by naloxone might indicate that the leucine form might have partial agonist (i.e., both agonist and antagonist) activity at opiate receptor sites, whereas met-enkephalin may be more of a true narcotic agonist. This is in contrast to the findings of Chang et al. (1976) in which they predict, on the basis of the sodium shift on opiate receptor binding [when binding is performed in the presence and absence of sodium pure agonists suffer 12- to 60-fold losses of inhibitory potency with the addition of sodium, antagonists exhibit onefold to threefold losses, and partial agonists have intermediate sodium response ratios (Pert and Snyder, 1974)], that met-enkephalin is a partial agonist and leu-enkephalin is a pure agonist.

Leu-enkephalin failed to produce significant changes in tail flock latencies over a wide range of doses (30–360 μg/rat) when infused into the PAG in rats in a study performed by Chang and co-workers (1976). In this study very high doses of met-enkephalin were necessary to produce a naloxone-reversible analgesic response. It is difficult to understand the lack of activity in this study, especially since the peptide was injected into one of the sites of morphine action (PAG). This finding with leu-enkephalin is in contrast to previous reports of analgesic activity following both intracerebral administration in the PAG (Malick and Goldstein, 1977) and intraventricular infusion (Belluzzi et al., 1976) in the rat tail flick test.

In summary, leu-enkephalin has benerally been shown to be an analgesic following both infusion into various areas of the brain, and in one case it even produced a weak, short-lasting antinociceptive response following intravenous administration. In general, with the exception of the results of Malick and Goldstein (1977) in which leu- and met-enkephalin were essentially equipotent, most investigators have reported the leu-enkephalin is less potent as an analgesic than the methionine form of enkephalin.

Beta-Endorphin

Beta-endorphin, the 31 amino acid fraction of β-lipotropin which contains within it the exact sequence of methionine-enkephalin (β-LPH 61-65), was first shown to be a potent analgesic by Loh et al. (1976). Doses of 0.5 and 1.0 μg intraventricularly to mice produced a dose-related analgesic response in both the hot plate and tail flick procedures. The analgesic action lasted from 60 to 90 minutes postinfusion and closely resembled the duration observed with morphine under similar conditions. Beta-endorphin (0.5 μg/mouse, i.c.v.) also produced a significant antinociceptive response in the acetic-acid-induced writhing test; the duration of this action was also 60–90 minutes (Loh et al., 1976). In this original report the investigators also pointed out that β-endorphin (0.25 and 1.0 μg/rat, i.c.) produces a significant dose-related analgesic response in the ice water-induced shaking test in rats following infusion into the PAG. In this test repetitive shaking movements are induced by immersion of anesthetized rats into ice water. Although this latter model certainly measures central opiate-like activity, it is difficult to see how it is a measure of analgesic activity if the animals are anesthetized. All of the aforementioned analgesic responses were readily antagonized by pretreatment with naloxone. The ED_{50} doses for β-endorphin were calculated to be 0.92, 1.52, and 2.32 nmoles/kg, i.c., in the writhing, tail flick, and hot plate tests, respectively; thus, on a molar basis β-endorphin was approximately 18–33 times as potent as morphine in the mouse (Loh et al., 1976).

Numerous investigators have reported that β-endorphin is a potent, long-acting analgesic in both mice and rats in the tail flick and hot plate procedures, and in the acetic acid-induced writhing test in mice (see Table 6) following infusion into the brain.

Several authors have also evaluated the analgesic potential of β-endorphin following intravenous administration: potent analgesic activity was observed in the tail flick test in mice (Tseng et al., 1976b; Li et al., 1977) and in the hot plate procedure in mice (Tseng et al., 1976b). In the tail flick procedure β-endorphin exhibited an ED_{50} of 3.3 μmoles/kg, i.v., and it was 3.4 times as potent as morphine (Li et al., 1977). The duration of β-endorphin's analgesic activity following intravenous infusion was between 20 and 30 minutes. In the studies by Tseng and associates (1976b) the duration of activity with β-endorphin was between 30 and 60 minutes postintravenous infusion (see Table 6).

Feldberg and Smyth (1976) demonstrated significant analgesic activity in the cat following infusion (i.c.v.) into the third ventricle. This activity was reported to last for more than two hours post-infusion as measured by a tail pinch procedure. Doses of β-endorphin as low as 2.5 μg, i.c.v., produced a weak but statistically significant analgesic response, whereas at higher doses (10–20 μg; 2.9–5.7 nmoles) potent long-lasting analgesia was observed. In these studies β-endorphin was estimated to be 100–200 times as potent as morphine.

Meglio and co-workers (1977) also evaluated β-endorphin as an analgesic in cats. In their pinch test they evaluated the responses of cats to pinching of the tail, ears, and limbs with forceps and to electrical stimulation of the tooth pulp prior to and following intraventricular infusion of drugs. Following infusion of 6.25 μg of β-endorphin, no significant alterations in behavior or responses to pain were observed. Although the 12.5-μg dose also failed to elicit analgesia, behavioral alterations (e.g., fine tremors, mild excitation) were seen. Significant analgesic activity was observed in both the pinch procedure and the tooth pulp test at both higher doses (25 and 50 μg, i.c.v.) of β-endorphin (Meglio et al., 1977). The analgesia produced by β-endorphin lasted for between two and

Table 6. Effects of β-Endorphin in Various Analgesic Tests

Investigator(s)	Species	Analgesic Model	Route of Administration	Dose (μg)	Injection Volume (μl)	Analgesic Activity
Feldberg and Smyth (1976)	Cat	Tail pinch	i.c.v.[a]	2.5–20	40	Significant analgesia at all doses; duration >2 hours
Graf et al. (1976)	Rat	Tail flick	i.c.v.	0.8 nmole	20	Potent analgesic activity; onset (15–30 minutes); duration (60–90 minutes)
Loh et al. (1976)	Mouse	Tail flick Hot plate Acetic acid Writhing	i.c.v.	0.5, 1	5	Dose related analgesia; duration (60–90 minutes)
	Rat	Ice water-induced shaking	i.c. (PAG)[b]	0.25, 1	0.5	Dose-related analgesia
Tseng et al. (1976a)	Mouse	Tail flick Hot plate	i.c.v.	Several[c]	5	ED_{50} = 0.15 μg/mouse; duration >60 minutes
Tseng et al. (1976b)	Mouse	Tail flick	i.v.[d]	8–20 mg/kg	—[e]	ED_{50} = 9.4 (6.9–12.8) mg/kg; duration (30–60 minutes)
	Mouse	Hot plate	i.v.	8–20 mg/kg	—	ED_{50} = 12.0 (8.0–18.0) mg/kg; duration (30–60 minutes)
Van Ree et al. (1976)	Rat	Hot plate (54.2°C)	i.c.v.	0.3–4.5	3	Significant analgesia only at 4.5 μg/rat; onset (20 minutes); duration (40–60 minutes)

Table 6 (Continued)

Bradbury et al. (1977)	Rat	Hot plate (55.5°C)	i.c.v.	0.0015 μmole	10	Potent analgesic activity; duration up to 100 minutes
Catlin et al. (1977)	Man	Cancer pain	i.v.	6.3, 100, 180 μg/kg	—[e]	One subject at each dose; significant analgesia at 6.3 and 180 μg/kg; very preliminary evaluation
Geisow et al. (1977)	Rat	Tail flick	i.c.v.	Several[c]	5	Significant analgesia between 0.6–1.6 nmoles/rat
Li et al. (1977)	Mouse	Tail flick	i.c.v.	Several[c]	—[e]	ED_{50} = 0.03 (0.02–0.04) nmole/mouse. Duration = 30–60 minutes; 48.4 times as potent as morphine
	Mouse	Hot plate	i.c.v.	Several[c]	—[e]	ED_{50} = 0.03 (0.02–0.04) nmole/mouse; 32.8 times as potent as morphine
	Mouse	Acetic acid writhing	i.c.v.	Several[c]	—[e]	ED_{50} = 0.02 (0.02–0.04) nmole/mouse; 17.3 times as potent as morphine
	Mouse	Tail flick	i.v.	Several[c]	—[e]	ED_{50} = 3.32 (1.86–5.69) μmoles/kg; 3.4 times as potent as morphine; duration = 20–30 minutes

Table 6 (Continued)

Investigator(s)	Species	Analgesic Model	Route of Administration	Dose (μg)	Injection Volume (μl)	Analgesic Activity
Meglio et al. (1977)	Cat	Pinch (tail, limbs, ears) Tooth pulp stimulation	i.c.v.	6.25–50	0.5 ml	Minimal effective dose = 25 μg; duration = 120–180 minutes
Roemer et al. (1977)	Mouse	Tail flick	i.c.v.	Several[c]	—[e]	ED_{50} = 0.3 μg/mouse
Szekely et al. (1977b)	Rat	Tail flick	i.c.v.	Several[c]	20	ED_{50} = 0.59 nmole/rat; duration = 60–120 minutes
Wei et al. (1977)	Mouse	Hot plate	i.c.v.	Several[c]	20	ED_{50} = 0.17 nmole/mouse
	Rat	Ice-water-induced shaking	i.c.v.[f]	Several[c]	1	Dose-related analgesia; ED_{50} = 0.4 nmole/rat
	Mouse	Tail flick	i.c.v.	Several[c]	5	ED_{50} = 0.03 nmole/mouse; 34.7 times as potent as morphine
Yamashiro et al. (1977)	Mouse	Tail flick	i.c.v.	Several[c]	5	ED_{50} = 0.11 μg/mouse
Hosobuchi and Li (1978)	Man	Heat	i.c.v.	100–400	2 ml	Pain relief for as long as 6 hours

[a] Intracerebroventricular
[b] Intracerebral; periaqueductal gray
[c] Actual doses not reported
[d] Intravenous
[e] Not reported
[f] Periaqueductal gray fourth ventricular space

three hours postinfusion. In their procedures, morphine sulfate failed to exhibit significant alterations in pain thresholds until doses of 150 and 200 µg were infused intraventricularly; thus β-endorphin was approximately six times as potent as morphine.

Because of its potent, long-lasting analgesic activity in animals, β-endorphin has been evaluated as an analgesic in humans. Catlin and associates (1977) were the first to evaluate the analgesic potential of β-endorphin in humans in a very preliminary manner in only three patients suffering with chronic pain as a result of advanced cancer. Of the three subjects evaluated, two exhibited a good analgesic response to β-endorphin (one each at doses of 6.3 and 180 µg/kg, i.v.) and one subject reported a slight reduction in pain following 100 µg/kg, i.v. Morphine (125 µg/kg, i.v.) produced good to excellent analgesic responses in all three subjects. As a result of this open trial, β-endorphin clearly appeared to be an analgesic in humans.

Hosobuchi and Li (1978) evaluated the analgesic potential of β-endorphin following intraventricular infusion in patients who had been implanted with electrodes for producing electrical brain stimulation-induced analgesia from the central gray. They administered total doses of 100, 200, and 400 µg, i.c.v., to three patients suffering from intractable pain that had only been managed with opiate analgesics. The minimal effective dose for producing a significant analgesic response was found to be 200 µg. Alterations of acute pain thresholds as measured by thermal dolorimetry were also observed; however, clinical pain relief occurred much sooner than and outlived the elevation of acute pain thresholds by four to six hours. The pain relief produced by β-endorphin was antagonized by intravenous infusion of 0.8 mg of naloxone (Hosobuchi and Li, 1978). This study, once again in a very small patient population, indicated that β-endorphin could produce a powerful, long-lasting analgesic action following intra ventricular administration; no adverse side effects were noted. Additional clinical trials with strict double-blind controls are necessary fully to evaluate the analgesic potential of β-endorphin in humans.

In summary, β-endorphin has been shown to be a potent, long-acting analgesic in rodents, cats, and people. In comparison with morphine, β-endorphin was found to be approximately 18–33 times as potent as this poppy derivative following intracerebroventricular administration in rodents and approximately three to four times as potent following intravenous infusion.

Beta-Lipotropin

Beta-lipotropin (β-LPH), a 91 amino acid peptide that may be a
prohormone (Lazarus et al., 1976) for some of the morphinomimetic
peptides (e.g., β-endorphin, met-enkephalin) also has been shown to
possess analgesic activity (Ronai et al., 1976). Ronai and associates
reported that β-LPH was approximately two times weaker than
morphine as an analgesic (calculated on a molar basis) following
intraventricular administration in the tail flick test in rats; ED_{50}
values were 7.7 and 17.0 nmoles/rat for morphine and β-LPH
respectively. In this study the analgesic activity of both β-LPH
and morphine peaked between 30 and 60 minutes and at the
highest doses lasted for up to 120 minutes postinfusion. Subcutaneous administration of naloxone (2 mg/kg) antagonized the
analgesic effects of both morphine and β-LPH. β-LPH was completely inactive as an analgesic when administered intravenously in
doses up to 130 mg/kg.

In contrast, Feldberg and Smyth (1977) failed to demonstrate
any analgesic activity with β-LPH (150 μg, i.c.v.) in the cat using
the tail pinch method of Russell and Tate (1975). In fact, they
failed to observe any morphine-like behavioral effects following
the infusion of β-LPH. In this same study doses of 10 and 20 μg
of β-endorphin produced a potent, long-lasting analgesic response.

Synthetic Endorphin Analogues

The purpose of this chapter is not to discuss the analgesic
activities of the multitude of synthetic endorphins that have been
synthesized in laboratories around the world. Only a very few
examples will be given of structural modifications that have suc-
ceeded in improving the analgesic potency of the naturally occurring peptides, presumably primarily by preventing their rapid
enzymatic catabolism.

The analgesic activity of met-enkephalin persists only for a few
minutes or so, even after infusion at sites in the brain where
morphine elicits analgesia for several hours. It has been discovered
that met-enkephalin's short duration of activity is attributable to
the fact that it is rapidly destroyed by brain enzymes. Pert and
co-workers (1976) concluded that the rapid loss of activity of
met-enkephalin was due to rapid cleavage of its Tyr^1-Gly^2 peptide
bond. Thus substitutions that protect this bond from cleavage
should produce longer-acting analgesic peptides. Indeed, substitu-

tion of met-enkephalinamide at the 2-position with D-alanine resulted in a pentapeptide that retained high affinity for opiate receptors and demonstrated high potency and a long duration of analgesic activity *in vivo* (Pert et al., 1976). [D-Ala^2]-met-enkephalinamide (10 μg/rat, i.c., PAG) produced significant increases in tail flick latencies that persisted for at least three hours postinfusion. Although the analgesic activity of 5 μg of morphine was more intense at one and two hours postinfusion, its duration of activity appeared to be about the same as observed with the synthetic enkephalin analogue. [D-Ala^2]-met-enkaphalinamide failed to cause analgesia up to 50 mg/kg, intravenously; this most likely was due to its failure to cross the blood–brain barrier. The activity of the [D-Ala^2] analogue could be significantly antagonized by pretreatment with naloxone (2 mg/kg, i.p.). These results have been confirmed and extended by Walker et al. (1977). They reported that [D-Ala^2]-met-enkephalin produced an antinociceptive response (tail flock) of greater magnitude, which lasted about 30 times longer than that produced by the naturally occurring met-enkephalin following intraventricular infusion in the rat.

Numerous analogues of both met- and leu-enkephalin have been synthesized. One of these, Try-D-Ala-Gly-Phe-D-Leu (Wellcome: BW 180C), exhibited greater antinociceptive potency than morphine, but was of shorter duration (Baxter et al., 1977). Dutta and associates (1977) synthesized approximately 200 enkephalin analogues and found that a few [e.g., Tyr-D-Ala-Gly-Phe-Leu-NH (CH$_2$)$_2$NHMe] even exhibited significant analgesic activity after intravenous doses as low as 5 mg/kg in the hot plate (56°C) test in mice. (D-Met^2, Pro^5)-enkephalinamide was found to be 5.5 times as potent as morphine following intravenous infusion (rat tail flock), and it was claimed to be the first peptide synthesized that was more potent than β-endorphin (Szekely et al., 1977b; Bajusz et al., 1977). Subsequently, several other enkephalin analogues were reported to be active even after oral administration in the mouse tail flock test (Roemer and Pless, 1979).

Roemer et al. (1977) synthesized a very interesting enkephalin analogue, [D-Ala^2,MePhe^4 Met-(O)^5-ol]-enkephalin (Sandoz: FK 33-824). Folliwing intraventricular administration (rat tail flock), compound FK 33-824 was found to be about 23, 1000, and 30,000 times as potent (on a molar basis) as β-endorphin, morphine, and met-enkephalin respectively. In addition, FK 33-824 was also reported to possess potent and prolonged analgesic activity after parenteral and even oral administration in rodents (Roemer et al., 1977). Following subcutaneous administration FK 33-824 was approximately twice as potent as morphine in mice (hot plate), as well as in rats (inflamed paw pressure test) (Randall and Selitto, 1957). Thirty minutes after oral administration FK 33-824 was approximately five (tail flick) and three and a half (hot plate) times as potent as morphine as an analgesic in mice. FK 33-824 exhibited remarkable stability compared with naturally occurring enkephalins and exhibited a duration of activity following intravenous administration of at least five hours in the rhesus monkey shock titration test. Compound FK 33-824 has been tested for analgesic potential in humans (Stacher et al., 1979) and has been shown to produce a significant increase in tolerance of electrically induced pain but virtually no change in pain thresholds after 1 mg, intramuscularly; morphine exhibits the same profile of activity in this procedure. Thus in humans, FK 33-824 mimicked the analgesic profile of morphine in very preliminary studies.

From the key examples that have been cited it should be evident that quite a few synthetic enkephalin analogues have been produced that are both more stable and more potent than the naturally occurring enkephalins.

TOLERANCE

Tseng and co-workers (1976a) attempted to learn whether the analgesic actions of β-endorphin would be likely to tolerate on repeated administration by determining whether it would exhibit cross-tolerance in rodents that had received chronic morphine. In this study mice were rendered tolerant to morphine by subcutaneously implanting them with morphine pellets for three days; controls were implanted with placebo pellets. The pellets were removed 72 hours after implantation and the mice were injected intracerebroventricularly with either β-endorphin or morphine, using the method of Haley and McCormick (1957). Analgesic activity was then assessed by utilizing both the tail flock and hot plate procedures. In placebo-implanted mice β-endorphin (1 μg/mouse, i.c.v.) produced a significant analgesic response in 80–100% of the mice tested in both analgesic models. However, in the morphine-pellet-implanted groups β-endorphin produced a significantly diminished analgesic response. When median antinociceptive doses were calculated, β-endorphin exhibited an eight- to ninefold increase in AD50 values in the morphine-implanted mice as compared with controls; morphine exhibited similar tolerance effects. Thus β-endorphin clearly exhibited analgesic cross-tolerance to morphine in mice.

In another study subacute administration of β-endorphin (4.5 μg/
rat, i.c.v., twice daily for two days and once on the test day) resulted
in the development of tolerance to its analgesic effects in the tail
flock procedure in rats (Van Ree et al., 1976). In addition, in
rats treated repeatedly with β-endorphin there was some evidence
of cross-tolerance to intracerebroventricularly administered
morphine. However, when morphine was administered intraperitoneally to animals that had received the same β-endorphin
treatment for three days, no signs of cross-tolerance were evident.
The only explanation given by the authors for this discrepancy was
that perhaps "the population of receptors involved in mediating
the antinociceptive effects of relatively low peripheral doses of
morphine may not be identical to that occupied after intracerebral
injection" (Van Ree et al., 1976).

In cats acute tolerance was observed to the analgesic effects of
β-endorphin if a second administration (i.c.v.) was given within 24
hours of the initial treatment (Meglio et al., 1977; Hosobuchi et
al., 1977). If the second administration of β-endorphin was given
48 hours or more after initial exposure, no tolerance was observed
(Hosobuchi et al., 1977). Although tolerance to the analgesic
actions of β-endorphin occurred very rapidly, the behavioral
syndrome (e.g., tremor, excitation, stereotypy) still persisted
(Hosobuchi et al., 1977). Hosobuchi and co-workers reported that
intraperitoneal injection of 5-hydroxytryptophan (10 mg/kg)
could reverse the tolerance to the analgesic activity of β-endorphin
as well as potentiate the analgesic effects of a subliminal dose of
β-endorphin. Thus their results suggested that perhaps β-endorphin
produces its analgesic effect by activation of serotonergic pathways.
Earlier reports (Contreras et al., 1973) demonstrated similar interactions between morphine and 5-hydroxytryptophan in that the
latter both reduced the development of tolerance to morphine and
potentiated its analgesic actions in mice.

In rats that have been made dependent upon and tolerant to
morphine (pellet implantation for five days) significantly elevated
brain enkephalin levels were observed (Simantov and Snyder,
1976). In addition, when these rats were treated with naloxone
(1 mg/kg, i.p.), enkephalin levels dropped to control levels within
one hour. Thus there appears to be an excellent correlation
between the development of tolerance to the analgesic effects of
morphine and elevated enkephalin levels.

Tolerance has also been observed at the neuronal level in
electrophysiologic studies. Briefly, opiates and endorphins have
been shown to decrease the sensitivity of single neurons to putative

excitatory transmitters and tolerance to these inhibitory actions
appears to develop following repeated exposure (Fry et al., 1978).

In summary, tolerance to the analgesic actions of β-endorphin
develops rapidly upon repeated administration and, although the
results are not as consistent, there also appears to be a cross-
tolerance between endorphins and morphine.

PHYSICAL DEPENDENCE AND ABUSE POTENTIAL

Wei and Loh (1976) were the first to demonstrate that the
endorphins could cause physical dependence. In order to show the
development of physical dependence in rats with substances that
are catabolized very rapidly (e.g., met-enkephalin), they used
osmotic minipumps for chronic drug delivery directly into the
brain via chronically indwelling cannulae (PAG—fourth ventricular
space). When rats that had been infused for 70 hours with met-
enkephalin or β-endorphin were challenged with naloxone, they
manifested a morphine-like withdrawal syndrome characterized
primarily by shaking, chattering of teeth, and repeated attempts to
escape (Wei and Loh, 1976; Loh et al., 1976). When seven
enkephalin analogues were evaluated (Wei, 1978), an excellent
correlation was found to exist between potency as an analgesic
and physical dependency liability; that is, the greater the antinociceptive activity, the greater the potential for producing physical
dependence. Thus endorphins clearly demonstrated physical
dependence liability in rats following subacute infusion directly
into the brain.

Schulz and Herz (1976) claimed to be able to predict dependence
liability with narcotics using an *in vitro* model, the isolated guinea
pig ileum. In their preparation myenteric plexus–longitudinal
muscle strips taken from morphine-tolerant/dependent guinea pigs,
which were kept in continuous contact with normorphine after
removal, exhibited tonic contracture upon naloxone challenge
("withdrawal response"). As a result of their evaluation in this
model it was predicted that both leu- and met-enkephalin would
exhibit morphine-like physical dependence.

At the neuronal level physical dependence liability can be
demonstrated by the naloxone-induced increases in spontaneous
and/or L-glutamate- and acetylcholine-induced activity observed in
single cell preparations from morphine-tolerant/dependent rats
(Fry et al., 1978); these enhanced responses appear to represent
specific withdrawal effects at the single neuron level.

Tseng and co-workers (1976a) used a modification of the mouse jump test (Way et al., 1969) to determine the physical dependence liability of β-endorphin. In this procedure mice were rendered morphine dependent by pellet implantation; 72 hours later the pellets were removed and the mice were challenged with naloxone and observed for the precipitation of withdrawal jumping. Beta-endorphin caused a dose-related inhibition of naloxone-induced jumping in morphine-tolerant mice; on a molar basis, β-endorphin was ten times more potent than morphine as a suppressant of jumping. In contrast to β-endorphin, met-enkephalin failed to inhibit jumping at doses up to 200 μg/mouse, i.c.v. Thus β-endorphin exhibited clear-cut physical dependence liability in the mouse jump test, a procedure considered to be a reliable predictor of such activity.

Self-administration procedures are used as a means of predicting substance abuse liability in humans. Belluzzi and Stein (1977) found that both met- and leu-enkephalin were self-administered by the rat. In these studies each lever press delivered 1 μl of the drug solution into the lateral ventricle via a chronically indwelling cannula. A subsequent study by Mello and Mendelson (1978) in rhesus monkeys clearly demonstrated that a potent, long-lasting synthetic enkephalin analogue, FK 33-824, was intravenously self-administered in both drug-naive and morphine-dependent animals. Thus all of the naturally occurring and synthetic endorphins that have been evaluated thus far would be predicted to possess significant abuse potential for humans.

Although elevated brain enkephalin levels were observed in rats treated chronically with morphine (Simantov and Snyder, 1976), no significant alteration in narcotic receptors, either in affinity or number of binding sites (ligands: ^{3}H-etorphine and ^{3}H-naltrexone), was observed in any brain area studied from rats that were implanted with morphine pellets for several days to yield a physically dependent/tolerant state (Bonnet et al., 1976). Thus the tolerance and physical dependence that occur after chronic administration of opiates is not due to obvious changes in opiate receptors in brain.

CONCLUSIONS

Endogenous modulation of pain is not a new concept. However, the discovery of the endorphins has given us the physiologic foundation for such beliefs. Clinical pain relief can be produced by several types of stimuli: acupuncture (Mayer et al., 1977); electrical brain stimulation (Adams, 1976; Richardson and Akil, 1973); transcutaneous electrical stimulation (Chapman and Benedetti, 1977); or by "counterirritation" with chemicals, pressure, or extreme temperatures (Gammon and Starr, 1941). It has been suggested that these responses may be the result of endorphin release or the activation of some endogenous antinociceptive processes.

Direct evidence that endorphins can modulate or control neuronal activity in neurons in the CNS that influences pain perception comes from iontophoretic studies. Endorphins have been shown to depress the evoked excitation caused by peripheral noxious stimulation in thalamic nociceptive neurons in rats (Hill and Pepper, 1978) and to reduce firing rates of nociceptive neurons in the trigeminal nucleus of cats (Anderson et al., 1978).

In patients suffering from chronic organic pain syndromes, significantly lower lumbar fluid endorphin levels have been observed (Almay et al., 1978). In another study in patients with intractable pain, electrical stimulation of periventricular brain sites caused a significant decrease in pain accompanied by a significant rise in ventricular enkephalin levels (Akil et al., 1978).

Thus there is strong evidence for the control or modulation of pain pathways by endorphins, and both the naturally occurring peptides and several more potent synthetic analogues have clearly been shown to be analgesics in both animals and humans. However, the endorphins that have been discovered to date do not appear to offer any advantages over existing poppy derivatives inasmuch as they exhibit tolerance, physical dependence liability, and cross-tolerance to morphine; produce respiratory depression (Florez and Mediavilla, 1977); and are self-administered by animals. As a result of these findings, it would be predicted that the endorphins evaluated thus far would exhibit a high degree of abuse liability in humans and cause the same types of side effects. Thus, unless some advantage other than potency can be discovered, it is highly unlikely that the endorphins will be used widely as antinociceptive agents in human beings.

SUMMARY

The first endogenous morphine-like substances that were discovered, leu- and met-enkephalin, have consistently been shown to be very short-acting analgesics in animals. In a few experiments in which the enkephalins were infused directly into brain sites (e.g., PAG) that have been proposed to be sites of action for morphine, the enkephalins have been shown to be nearly as potent as morphine itself. However, the enkephalins have generally appeared to be weak in comparison with morphine because they usually have been infused into the ventricles and most of their activity has been lost during diffusion to active sites as a result of rapid enzymatic degradation. In general, the enkephalins are inactive as analgesics following intravenous administration.

In contrast to the enkephalins, β-endorphin has been found to be a very potent analgesic following both intracerebral and intravenous administration in animals. Beta-endorphin has consistently been shown to be more potent than morphine, and it exhibits a long duration of analgesic activity. It also has been reported to exhibit significant antinociceptive activity in humans. Several enkephalin analogues (e.g., FK 33-824) have also been shown to be potent, long-lasting analgesics.

Tolerance to the analgesic actions of the endorphins develops rapidly following repeated administration and they produce physical dependence in laboratory animals. The endorphins exhibit all of the side effects of the poppy derivatives (e.g., constipation, respiratory depression) and appear to possess a high degree of abuse potential as demonstrated by the fact that they are self-administered by rats and monkeys. Although there is little doubt that endorphinergic pathways modulate or control pain perception, the compounds that have been discovered to date offer no advantages over the narcotics available today, with the possible exception of potency.

REFERENCES

Adams, J. E. Naloxone reversal of analgesia produced by brain stimulation in the human. *Pain* 1976; 2:161-166.

Akil, H., Mayer, D. J., and Liebeskind, J. C. Antagonism of stimulation produced analgesia by naloxone, a narcotic antagonist. *Science* 1976; 191:961-962.

Akil, H., Richardson, D. E., Hughes, J., and Barchas, J. D. Enkephalin like material elevated in ventricular cerebrospinal fluid of pain patients after analgetic focal stimulation. *Science* 1978; 201:463-465.

Almay, B. G. L., Johansson, F., vonKnorring, L., et al. Endorphins in chronic pain. I. Differences in CSF endorphin levels between organic and psychogenic pain syndromes. *Pain* 1978; 5:153-162.

Anderson, R. K., Lund, J. P., and Puil, E. Enkephalin and substance P effects related to trigeminal pain. *Can. J. Physiol. Pharmacol.* 1978; 56:216-222.

Balagura, S., and Ralph, T. The analgesic effect of electrical stimulation of the diencephalon and mesencephalon. *Brain Res.* 1973; 60:369-381.

Bajusz, S., Ronai, A. Z., Szekely, J. I., et al. A superactive antinociceptive pentapeptide, (D-Met^2, Pro^5)-enkephalinamide. *FEBS Letters* 1977; 76:91-92.

Baxter, M. G., Goff, D., Miller, A. A., and Saunders, I. A. Effect of a potent synthetic opioid pentapeptide in some antinociceptive and behavioural tests in mice and rats. *Br. J. Pharmacol.* 1977; 59:455-456.

Belluzzi, J. D., and Stein, L. Enkephalin may mediate euphoria and drive-reduction reward. *Nature* 1977; 266:556-558.

Belluzzi, J. D., Grant, N., Garsky, V., et al. Analgesia induced *in vivo* by central administration of enkephalin in the rat. *Nature* 1976; 260: 625-626.

Bloom, A. S., Dewey, W. L., Harris, L. S., et al. The correlation between antinociceptive activity of narcotics and their antagonists as measured in the mouse tail flick test and increased synthesis of brain catecholamines. *J. Pharmacol. Exp. Ther.* 1976; 198:33-41.

Bonnet, K. A., Hiller, J. M., and Simon, E. J. (1976): The effects of chronic opiate treatment and social isolation on opiate receptors in the rodent brain. *In* H. Kosterlitz (Ed.), *Opiates and Endogenous Opioid Peptides*. New York: North-Holland Publishing Co., pp. 335-343.

Bradbury, A. F., Smyth, D. G., Snell, C. R., et al. C-fragment of lipotropin has a high affinity for brain opiate receptors. *Nature* 1976; 260: 793-795.

Bradbury, A. F., Smyth, D. G., Snell, C. R., et al. Comparison of the analgesic properties of lipotropin C-fragment and stabilized enkephalins in the rat. *Biochem. Biophys. Res. Communs.* 1977; 74:748-754.

Brittain, R. T., Lehrer, D. N., and Spencer, P. S. Phenylquinone writhing test: Interpretation of data. *Nature* 1963; (London) 200:895-896.

Büscher, H. H., Hill, R. C., Romer, D., et al. Evidence for analgesic activity of enkephalin in the mouse. *Nature* 1976; 261:423-425.

Catlin, D. H., Hui, K. K., Loh, H. H., and Li, C. H. Pharmacologic activity of β-endorphin in man. *Commun. Psychopharmacol.* 1977; 1:493-500.

Chang, J. K., Fong, B. T. W., Pert, A., and Pert, C. B. Opiate receptor affinities and behavioral effects of enkephalin: Structure-activity relationship of ten synthetic peptide analogues. *Life Sci.* 1976; 18: 1473-1482.

Chapman, C. R., and Benedetti, C. Analgesia following transcutaneous electrical stimulation and its partial reversal by a narcotic antagonist. *Life Sci.* 1977; 21:1645-1648.

Chernov, H. I., Wilson, D. E., Fowler, F., and Plummer, A. J. Non-specificity of the mouse writhing test. *Arch. Int. Pharmacodyn. Ther.* 1967; 167:171-178.

Cochin, J. (1968). Methods for the appraisal of analgesic drugs for addiction liability. *In* A. Burger (Ed.), *Selected Pharmacological Testing Methods*, Vol. 3. New York: Marcel Dekker, Inc., pp. 121-169.

Contreras, E., Tomayo, L., Quijada, L., and Silva, E. Decrease of tolerance development to morphine by 5-hydroxytryptophan and some related drugs. *Europ. J. Pharmacol.* 1973; 22:339-343.

Cox, B. M., Goldstein, A., and Li, C. H. Opioid activity of a peptide [β-LPH-(61-91)], derived from β-lipotropin. *Proc. Nat. Acad. Sci. U.S.A.* 1976. 73 1821-1823.

D'Amour, F. E., and Smith, D. L. A method for determining loss of pain sensation. *J. Pharmacol. Exp. Ther.* 1941; 72:74-79.

Dewey, W. L., and Harris, L. S. Antinociceptive activity of the narcotic antagonist analgesics and antagonistic activity of narcotic analgesics in rodents. *J. Pharmacol. Exp. Ther.* 1971; 179:652-659.

Dutta, A. S., Gormley, J. J., Hayward, C. F., et al. Enkephalin analogues eliciting analgesia after intravenous injection. *Life Sci.* 1977; 21: 559-562.

Eddy, N. B., and Leimbach, D. Synthetic analgesics. II. Dithienylbutenyl- and dithienybutylamines. *J. Pharmacol. Exp. Ther.* 1953; 107:385-393.

Feldberg, W., and Smyth, D. G. The C-fragment of lipotropin—A potent analgesic. *J. Physiol.* 1976; 260:30P-31P.

Feldberg, W., and Smyth, D. G. C-fragment of lipotropin—An endogenous potent analgesic peptide. *Br. J. Pharmacol.* 1977; 60:445-453.

Fraser, H. F., and Harris, L. S. Narcotic and narcotic antagonist analgesics. *Ann. Rev. Pharmacol.* 1967; 7:277-300.

Fry, J. P., Zieglgansberger, W., and Herz, A. (1978): Single neurone studies of opiate tolerance and dependence. *In* J. M. vanRee and L. Terenius (Eds.), *Characteristics and Functions of Opioids.* New York: Elsevier/ North-Holland Biomedical Press, pp. 99-100.

Gammon, G. D., and Starr, I., Jr. Studies on the relief of pain by counter- irritation. *J. Clin. Invest.* 1941; 20:13-20.

Geisow, M. J., Deakin, J. F. W., Dostrovsky, J. O., and Smyth, D. G. Analgesic activity of lipotropin C fragment depends on carboxyl terminal tetrapeptide. *Nature* 1977; 269:167-168.

Goldstein, A. Opioid peptides (endorphins) in pituitary and brain. *Science* 1976; 193:1081-1086.

Goldstein, A., Lowney, L. I., and Pal, B. K. Stereospecific and nonspecific interactions of the morphine congener levorphanol in subcellular fractions of mouse brain. *Proc. Nat. Acad. Sci. U.S.A.* 1971; 68: 1742-1747.

Goldstein, A., Pryor, G. T., Otis, L. S., and Larsen, F. On the role of endogenous opioid peptides: Failure of naloxone to influence shock escape thresholds in the rat. *Life Sci.* 1976; 18:599-604.

Goldstein, J. M., and Malick, J. B. Lack of analgesic activity of substance P following intraperitoneal administration. *Life Sci.* 1969; 25:431-436.

Goodman, S. J., and Holcombe, V. (1976): Selective and prolonged analgesia in monkey resulting from brain stimulation. *In* J. J. Bonica and D. G. Albe-Fessard (Eds.), *Advances in Pain Research and Therapy*, Vol. 1, Proceedings of the First World Congress. New York: Raven Press, pp. 495-502.

Graf, L., Szekely, J. I., Ronai, A. Z., et al. Comparative study on analgesic effect of met[5]-enkephalin and related lipotropin fragments. *Nature* 1976; 263:240-242.

Haley, T. J., and McCormick, W. G. Pharmacological effects produced by intracerebral injection of drugs in the conscious mouse. *Br. J. Pharmacol.* 1957; 12:12-15.

Hambrook, J. M., Morgan, F. A., Rance, M. J., and Smith, C. F. C. Mode of deactivation of the enkephalins by rat and human plasma and rat brain homogenates. *Nature* 1976; 262:782-783.

Herz, A., Albus, K., Metys, J., et al. On the central sites for the anti- nociceptive action of morphine and fentamyl. *Neuropharmacology* 1970; 9:539-551.

Hill, R. G., and Pepper, C. M. The depression of thalamic nociceptive neurons by D-Ala^2, D-Leu^5-enkephalin. *Europ. J. Pharmacol.* 1978; 47:223-225.

Hosobuchi, Y., and Li, C. H. The analgesic activity of human β-endorphin in man. *Commun. Psychopharmacology* 1978; 2:33-37.

Hosobuchi, Y., Meglio, M., Adams, J. E., and Li, C. H. β-endorphin: Development of tolerance and its reversal by 5-hydroxytryptophan in cats. *Proc. Nat. Acad. Sci. U.S.A.* 1977; 74:4017-4019.

Hughes, J. Isolation of an endogenous compound from the brain with pharmacological properties similar to morphine. *Brain Res.* 1975; 88:295-308.

Hughes, J., Smith, T. W., Kosterlitz, H. W., et al. Identification of two related pentapeptides from the brain with potent opiate agonist activity. *Nature* 1975; 258:577-579.

Johannesson, T., and Woods, L. A. Analgesic action and brain and plasma levels of morphine and codeine in morphine tolerant, codeine tolerant and non-tolerant rats. *Acta Pharmacol. Toxicol.* 1964; 21:381-396.

Lazarus, L. H., Ling, N., and Guillemin, R. β-lipotropin as a prohormone for the morphinomimetic peptides and enkephalins. *Proc. Nat. Acad. Sci. U.S.A.* 1976; 73:2156-2159.

Leybin, L., Pinsky, C., LaBella, F. S., Havlicek, V., and Rezek, M. Intraventricular met^5-enkephalin causes unexpected lowering of pain threshold and narcotic withdrawal signs in rats. *Nature* 1976; 264: 458-459.

Li, C. H., Yamashiro, D., Tseng, L. F., and Loh, H. H. Synthesis and analgesic activity of human β-endorphin. *J. Med. Chem.* 1977; 20: 325-328.

Liebeskind, J. C., Guilbaud, G., Besson, J. M., and Oliveras, J. L. Analgesia from electrical stimulation of the periaqueductal gray matter in the cat: Behavioral observations and inhibitory effects on spinal cord interneurons. *Brain Res.* 1973; 50:441-446.

Ling, N., and Guillemin, R. Morphino-mimetic activity of synthetic fragments of β-lipotropin and analogs. *Proc. Nat. Acad. Sci. U.S.A.* 1976; 73: 3308-3310.

Ling, N., Burgus, R., and Guillemin, R. Isolation, primary structure, and synthesis of α-endorphin and γ-endorphin, two peptides of hypothalamic-hypophysial origin with morphinomimetic activity. *Proc. Nat. Acad. Sci. U.S.A.* 1976; 73:3942-3946.

Litchfield, J. T., Jr., and Wilcoxon, F. A simplified method of evaluating dose-effect experiments. *J. Pharmac. Exp. Ther.* 1949; 96:99-113.

Loh, H. H., Tseng, L. F., Wei, E., and Li, C. H. β-endorphin is a potent analgesic agent. *Proc. Nat. Acad. Sci. U.S.A.* 1976; 73:2895-2898.

Malick, J. B., and Goldstein, J. M. Analgesia following intracerebral administration of enkephalin in the rat. *Pharmacologist* 1976; 18:120.

Malick, J. B., and Goldstein, J. M. Analgesic activity of enkephalins following intracerebral administration in the rat. *Life Sci.* 1977; 20:827-832.

Mayer, D. J., and Hayes, R. Stimulation-produced analgesia: Development of tolerance and cross-tolerance to morphine. *Science* 1975; 188: 941-943.

Mayer, D. J., and Liebeskind, J. C. Pain reduction by focal electrical stimulation of the brain: An anatomical and behavioral analysis. *Brain Res.* 1974; 68:73-93.

Mayer, D. J., and Murphin, R. Stimulation-produced analgesia (SPA) and morphine analgesia (MA): Cross-tolerance from application at the same brain site. *Fed. Proc.* 1976; 35:385.

Mayer, D. J., and Price, D. D. Central nervous system mechanisms of analgesia. *Pain* 1976; 2:379-404.

Mayer, D. J., Price, D. D., and Rafii, A. Antagonism of acupuncture analgesia in man by the narcotic antagonist naloxone. *Brain Res.* 1977; 121:368-372.

Meglio, M., Hobobuchi, Y., Loh, H. H., et al. β-endorphin: Behavioral and analgesic activity in cats. *Proc. Nat. Acad. Sci. U.S.A.* 1977; 74: 774-776.

Mello, N. K., and Mendelson, J. H. Self-administration of an enkephalin analog by rhesus monkey. *Pharmacol. Biochem. Behav.* 1978; 9:579-586.

Oliveras, J. L., Besson, J. M., Guilaud, G., and Liebeskind, J. C. Behavioral and electrophysiological evidence of pain inhibition from midbrain stimulation in the cat. *Exp. Brain Res.* 1974; 20:32-44.

Pert, A., and Yaksh, T. Sites of morphine induced analgesia in the primate brain: Relation to pain pathways. *Brain Res.* 1974; 80:135-140.

Pert, C. B., and Snyder, S. H. Opiate receptors: Demonstration in nervous tissue. *Science* 1973; 179:1011-1014.

Pert, C. B., and Snyder, S. H. Opiate receptor binding of agonists and antagonists affected differentially by sodium. *Molec. Pharm.* 1974; 10:868-879.

Pert, C. B., Pert, A., Chang, J. K., and Fong, B. T. W. [D-Ala^2]-met-enkephalinamide: A potent, long-lasting synthetic pentapeptide analgesic. *Science* 1976; 194:330-332.

Randall, L. O., and Selitto, J. J. A method for measurement of analgesic activity on inflamed tissue. *Arch. Int. Pharmacodynam.* 1957; 111: 409-419.

Reynolds, D. V. Surgery in the rat during electrical analgesia induced by focal brain stimulation. *Science* 1969; 164:444-445.

Richardson, D. E., and Akil, H. (1973): Acute relief of intractable pain by brain stimulation in human patients. Paper presented at Annual Meeting of the American Association of Neurological Surgeons.

Roemer, D., and Pless, J. Structure activity relationship of orally active enkephalin analogues as analgesics. *Life Sci.* 1979; 24:621-624.

Roemer, D., Buescher, H. H., Hill, R. C., et al. A synthetic enkephalin analogue with prolonged parenteral and oral analgesic activity. *Nature* 1977; 268:547-549.

Ronai, A. Z., Szekely, J. I., Graf, L., Dunai-Kovacs, Z., and Bajusz, S. Morphine-like analgesic effect of a pituitary hormone, β-lipotropin. Life Sci. 1976; 19:733-738.

Russell, W. J., and Tate, M. A. A device for applying nociceptive stimulation by pressure. *J. Physiol.* (London) 1975; 248:5-7.

Schulz, R., and Herz, A. (1976): The guinea pig ileum as an *in vitro* model to analyze dependence liability of narcotic drugs. *In* H. Kosterlitz (Ed.), *Opiates and Endogenous Opioid Peptides.* New York: North-Holland Publishing Co., pp. 319-326.

Simantov, R., and Snyder, S. H. Elevated levels of enkephalin in morphine-dependent rats. *Nature* 1976; 262:505-507.

Simon, E. J., Hiller, J. M., and Edelman, I. Stereospecific binding of the potent narcotic analgesic [³H]etorphine to rat brain homogenate. *Proc. Nat. Acad. Sci. U.S.A.* 1973; 70:1947-1949.

Stacher, G., Bauer, P., Steinringer, H., et al. Effects of the synthetic enkephalin analogue FK 33-824 on pain threshold and pain tolerance in man. *Pain* 1979; 7:159-172.

Szekely, J. I., Ronai, A. Z., Dunai-Kovacs, et al. C-terminal fragment (residues 61-91) of β-lipotropin: Is it the natural opiate-like neurohormone of the brain? *Experientia* 1977; 33:54-55.

Szekely, J. I., Ronai, A. Z., Dunai-Kovacs, Z., et al. (D-Met²-Pro⁵)—enkephalinamide: A potent morphine-like analgesic. *Europ. J. Pharmacol.* 1977; 43:293-294.

Taber, R. I., Greenhouse, D. D., Rendell, J. K., and Irwin, S. Agonist and antagonist interactions of opioids on acetic acid induced stretching in mice. *J. Pharmacol. Exp. Ther.* 1969; 169:29-38.

Terenius, L. Stereospecific interaction between narcotic analgesics and a synaptic plasma membrane fraction of rat cerebral cortex. *Acta Pharmacol. Toxicol.* 1973; 32:317-321.

Tseng, L., Loh, H. H., and Li, C. H. β-endorphin: Cross-tolerance to and cross physical dependence on morphine. *Proc. Nat. Acad. Sci. U.S.A.* 1976; 73:4187-4189.

Tseng, L. F., Loh, H. H., and Li, C. H. β-endorphin: As a potent analgesic by intravenous injection. *Nature* 1976; 263:239-240.

Urca, G., Frenk, H., Liebeskind, J. C., and Taylor, A. N. Morphine and enkephalin: Analgesic and epileptic properties. *Science* 1977; 197: 83-86.

Van Ree, J. M., De Wied, D., Bradbury, A. F., et al. Induction of tolerance to the analgesic action of lipotropin C-fragment. *Nature* 1976; 264: 792-794.

Walker, J. M., Berntson, G. G., Sandman, C. A., et al. An analog of enkephalin having prolonged opiate-like effects *in vivo*. *Science* 1977; 196:85-87.

Way, E. L., Loh, H. H., and Shen, F. H. Simultaneous quantitative assessment of morphine tolerance and physical dependence. *J. Pharmacol. Exp. Ther.* 1969; 167:1-8.

Wei, E. (1978): Enkephalin analogs: Correlation of potencies for analgesia and physical dependence. *In* J. M. Van Ree and L. T. Terenius (Eds.), *Characteristics and Functions of Opioids.* New York: Elsevier/North-Holland Biomedical Press, pp. 445-446.

Wei, E., and Loh, H. (1976): Chronic, intracerebral infusion of morphine and peptides with osmotic minipumps and the development of physical dependence. *In* H. W. Kosterlitz (Ed.), *Opiates and Endogenous Opioid Peptides.* New York: North-Holland Publishing Co., pp. 303-310.

Wei, E. T., Tseng, L. F., Loh, H. H., and Li, C. H. Comparison of the behavioral effects of β-endorphin and enkephalin analogs. *Life Sci.* 1977; 21:321-328.

Yaksh, T. L., DuChateau, J. C., and Rudy, T. A. Antagonism by methysergide and cinanserin of the antinociceptive action of morphine administered into the periaqueductal gray. *Brain Res.* 1976; 104: 367-372.

Yamashiro, D., Tseng, L. F., Doneen, B. A., et al. β-endorphin: synthesis and morphine-like activity of analogs with D-amino acid residues in positions 1, 2, 4 and 5. *Int. J. Peptide Protein Res.* 1977; 10:159-166.

2

Extrapituitary Functions of Thyrotropin-Releasing Hormone

MICHAEL D. HIRSCH

Thyrotropin-releasing hormone (TRH) was the first and smallest hypothalamic polypeptide to be isolated, purified, characterized, and synthesized (Vale and Rivier, 1975; Vale et al., 1977); its sequential tripeptide-amino acid structure is L-pyroglutamyl-L-histidyl-L-proline amide (pGlu-His-Pro-NH$_2$). Synthetic TRH has been shown to stimulate *in vivo* and *in vitro* secretion of thyroid-stimulating hormones (TSH) from the adenohypophysis in all mammals (including humans). It effects prolactin (PRL) release as well (Brownstein, 1978; Vale and Rivier, 1975; Vale et al., 1977). Competitive radioreceptor TRH binding studies utilizing synthetic tritiated TRH ([^{3}H]-TRH) in pituitary tissues (mouse thyrotropic and rat somatotropic/prolactotropic tumor, as well as normal bovine and rat membrane preparations) reveal high specificity of binding: [^{3}H]-TRH binding is saturable; unlabeled TRH is capable of stoichiometric competition; and the majority of binding sites are localized in the plasma membrane subcellular fraction, which displays an approximate 40-fold increase in [^{3}H]-TRH binding when compared with the total adenohypophyseal homogenate (Burt and Snyder, 1975; Burt and Taylor, 1980; Grant et al., 1973; Labrie et al., 1972, 1978; Poirier et al., 1972). In addition, a large number of synthetic TRH structural analogues have been synthesized and studied in the pituitary (Burt and Snyder, 1975; Burt and Taylor, 1980; Grant et al., 1973; Vale et al., 1973, 1977; Vale and Rivier, 1975; Vale, Rivier and Burgus,

1971). In general, the relative *in vivo* biological potency
(percentage TSH release; percentage PRL release) of these
analogues correlates fairly well with their *in vitro* radioreceptor
[^{3}H]-TRH competitive binding capabilities (relative affinities) in
pituitary membrane receptors. Potent receptor antagonists, mainly
TRH analogues, capable of blocking TRH-stimulated release of TSH
have been synthesized (Bowers et al., 1976; Lybeck et al., 1973;
Sievertsson et al., 1975).

It has recently been found that hypothalamo-adenohypophyseal
oligopeptide hormones ("factors") act in the CNS quite differently
from their traditional endocrine-regulatory functions (Barbeau et
al., 1976; Cooper et al., 1978; Guillemin, 1978; Harris et al.,
1966; Hughes, 1978; Martin et al., 1975; Sandman et al., 1976;
Vale and Rivier, 1975; Vale et al., 1977). In support of Pearse's
amine precursor uptake and decarboxylation theory (APUD),
which postulates that all peptide-producing cells are derived from
the embryonal neuroectoderm (Pearse, 1978), Leppäluoto and
associates (1978), using RIA techniques, found TRH localized in
rat CNS, endocrine, and gastrointestinal (GI) tract tissues. Further,
a large series of studies indicate that TRH can antagonize
barbiturate-induced narcosis in the mouse. Of the several known
characteristics of this endogenous hypothalamic polypeptide
hormone, this specific behavioral effect is one of the most potent
and reliable cited (Prange et al., 1978a, 1978b). In addition to
mice, this analeptic effect has been demonstrated in several other
species. This chapter will be directed toward further elucidating
the possible central mechanisms of the TRH analeptic effect on
five levels: (1) physicochemical, (2) neurochemical, (3) physiologic,
(4) psychopharmacologic, and (5) behavioral.

The strength and significance of research related to TRH's
central activities are based upon several important parallel neuropeptide paradigms currently under investigation. These paradigms
can be generally classified as opioid peptides, adrenocorticotropic-
like peptides, and clinical adjuvants:

1. It has recently been found that five endogenous peptides—
met- and leu-enkephalin, and α-, β-, and γ-endorphin—have specific
receptors, and *in vivo* and *in vitro* "morphine-like" biological
properties in the CNS (Guillemin et al., 1976; Hughes, 1975;
Hughes et al., 1975; Lazarus et al., 1976). Their amino acid
sequences were initially characterized as fragments of the larger
β-lipotropin (β-LPH) pituitary hormone (Hughes et al., 1975),
although more recent evidence strongly indicate a biosynthetic
pathway for the enkephalins completely separate from that of
β-endorphin (Lewis et al., 1980). Radioreceptor and

radioimmunoassay (RIA) results reveal that the enkephalins are widely distributed throughout the CNS in high concentrations and have been located within the cerebral cortex, caudate nucleus, hypothalamus, thalamus, and posterior pituitary (Pollard et al., 1977; Simantov and Snyder, 1976; Snyder et al., 1978). Brain opioid receptors have a high affinity for enkephalins and a low affinity for β-endorphin; the neurohypophysis displays a reversed affinity relationship in this regard (Simantov and Snyder, 1977). Endogenous and synthetic opioid peptides have been implicated in direct neuromodulation (Barker et al., 1978), as well as in the central modulation of analgesia (Bloom et al., 1976; Haigler and Spring, 1978; Jacquet and Marks, 1976; Pert et al., 1977); sedation, immobility, hyperactivity-hyperreactivity, and catalepsy (Bloom et al., 1976; Browne and Segal, 1980; Chang et al., 1976; Goldstein et al., 1979; Haigler and Spring, 1978; Jacquet and Marks, 1976; Pert et al., 1977); learning and memory (Rigter, 1978); altered thermoregulation (Bloom et al., 1976); altered electrical self-stimulation activities (Van Ree and Otte, 1980); altered eating and grooming activities (Katz, 1980); and the attenuation of nociceptive responses during pregnancy (Gintzler, 1980).

These endogenous opioids are highly active in the opiate-twitch inhibition bioassay as well as the [^{3}H]-etorphine radioreceptor assay (Chang et al., 1976; Goldstein, 1976); there is a very high correlation between opioid peptide-induced analgesia and activities in both the bioassay (Kosterlitz and Waterfield, 1975) and the radioreceptor assay (Creese and Snyder, 1975; Chang et al., 1976). It also appears that the brain has a potent neuromodulatory mechanism for controlling central opioid actions (Jacquet et al., 1978).

2. The second major area of neuropeptide research stems from the recent discovery that structural modifications of amino acid sequences in parent and fragmentary analogues of adrenocorticotropic hormone (ACTH) and α- and β-melanocyte stimulating hormone (MSH)—structurally related to β-LPH—can lead to profound behavioral changes independent of classical endocrine actions (De Wied, 1974; Van Riezen et al., 1977). Recent findings suggest that a vascular route conveys ACTH from the pituitary directly to the brain (Bergland et al., 1980). Autoradiographic studies of the regional peptide distribution in the rat brain following intraventricular (i.vt.) [^{3}H]-ACTH$_{4-9}$ administrations reveal that these peptides may be acting preferentially upon a morphologically and functionally distinct class of brain neurons: 5 minutes after administration labeled cells were identified in the choroid plexus

of the lateral ventricles, lateral septal nucleus, caudate-putamen
region, stria terminalis, and cerebral cortex near the cannula tract
(Rees et al., 1980); 30 minutes after administration, other areas
were involved, including the hypothalamus, thalamus, fornix,
hippocampus, diagonal band of Broca, and habenular. ACTH,
MSH, and related structural analogues can restore impaired
acquisition of shuttle box avoidance behavior in hypophysectomized
rats (De Wied, 1974).

The behaviorally active core of ACTH is located in the N-terminal
amino acid sequence—$ACTH_{4-10}$—which is also present in α-MSH,
β-MSH, and β-LPH (De Wied, 1974, 1978; Urban and De Wied,
1976; Van Riezen et al., 1977). The general findings implicate
ACTH and structural analogues in motivational processes, learning,
and memory retrieval: Administration of these neuropeptides to
animals inhibits extinction of shuttle box and passive avoidance
responses, and food- and sex-motivated behaviors (De Wied, 1974;
Flood et al., 1976; Rigter et al., 1976; Urban and De Wied, 1976;
Wimersma Greidanus and De Wied, 1976; Van Riezen et al., 1977).
Low parenteral doses of $ACTH_{4-10}$ to sham operated rats delay
extinction of a conditioned avoidance response; however, higher
doses are ineffective in this paradigm when administered to rats
bearing extensive bilateral anterodorsal hippocampal lesions. This
suggests that intact limbic structures—including the hippocampus,
septum, and thalamic reticular nucleus—are required for neuropeptides to be efficacious (Wimersma Greidanus and De Wied,
1976). It has also been reported that parenteral administrations
of $ACTH/MSH_{4-10}$ profoundly enhance attention, visual-motor
learning, and visual memory in normal humans (Miller et al., 1976).

3. Endogenous and synthetic polypeptide analogues are
currently being investigated as adjuvants for clinical psychopharmacologic treatment regimes as well as possible etiological
factors in psychopathologic states: TRH produces an immediate
antidepressant effect in depressive patients (Ehrensing and Kastin,
1976; Prange and Wilson, 1972). This peptide is also an effective
potentiator in the L-Dopa (3,4-dihydroxyphenylalanine) plus
pargyline drug screening test (Plotnikoff et al., 1977); and it also
antagonizes α-methyl-p-tyrosine (AMPT, a tyrosine hydroxylase
inhibitor) induced depressions of spontaneous locomotor and
conditioned avoidance activities in rats (Kulig, 1975). It has been
reported that the peptide reduces schizophrenics' hallucinations
while improving their general psychiatric profiles (Wilson et al.,
1973). It has been suggested that the endogenous opioid peptides
play an important etiologic role in mental illness through their
actions upon homeostatic regulatory functions (Bloom et al.,

1976), and through an induction of catatonia (Bloom et al., 1976; Jacquet and Marks, 1976). Roubicek and colleagues (1980) reported that parenteral injections of synthetic met-enkephalin produced transient improvements in the symptomology of endogenous depressives and hebephrenic schizophrenics.

Tentative results indicate that acupuncture-induced analgesia may be related to endorphin activities (Pomeranz, 1977). Ho and co-workers (1980) report that heroin addicts have diminished β-endorphin levels, suggestive of disrupted pituitary endorphin systems in these patients. $ACTH_{4-10}$ administrations have been shown to enhance profoundly dimensional attention in mentally retarded subjects (Ferris et al., 1976). It also improves attention in normal subjects (Miller et al., 1976). Clinical studies indicate that this neuropeptide is a relatively safe drug in humans and animals (Van Riezen et al., 1977). Gold and colleagues (1981) report that intranasal infusions of a synthetic vasopression analogue improve cognitive functions and ameliorate the symptomology of depressive patients. Clinical trials indicate that luteinizing hormone-releasing hormone (LHRH) may increase the libidinal drive of hypogonadal men (Mortimer et al., 1974).

TRH Antagonism of Barbiturate Narcosis

Prange and colleagues (1974) found that TRH has very potent and significant antagonist capabilities in rodents (mice and rats) for barbiturate-induced narcosis (indices: righting reflex; activity departing a circle) and hypothermia. These findings have been reliably confirmed and further extended (Bissette et al., 1976; Breese et al., 1974a, 1974b, 1975; Cohn et al., 1976; Crowley and Hydinger, 1976, 1977; Holaday et al., 1978; Kalivas and Horita, 1979, 1980; Prange et al., 1974, 1975, 1978a, 1978b). The TRH analeptic effect has been found to vary with both TRH and barbiturate dosage levels, with route of TRH administration [intraperitoneal (i.p.), intramuscular (i.m.), intravenous (i.v.), intracisternal (i.c.), intracerebral (i.cb.), and intraventricular (i.vt.)], and with drug order and interinjection durations. This effect is independent of the classical pituitary-thyroid axis [it is unaffected by hypophysectomy, and L-triiodothyronine (T_3) or thyroid-stimulating hormone (TSH, thyrotropin) administrations]. The analeptic effect can be dissociated from thermoregulatory actions; it also occurs for a wide range of barbiturates (pento-barbital, phenobarbital, thiopental, secobarbital, and amobarbital), as well as a number of structurally different sedative-hypnotics (chloral hydrate, reserpine, chlorpromazine, diazepam, and ethanol). TRH does not affect barbiturate metabolism [(^{3}H)-pentobarbital disposition]. The TRH analeptic effect has been further extended to other species (mice, rats, hamsters, gerbils, guinea pigs, rabbits, and monkeys) and appears to be non-sex related (at least in mice receiving i.p. drug administrations of TRH and barbiturate).

Critical Issues

Several important features of the TRH analeptic effect need to be further clarified.

1. Since the effect occurs independently of the pituitary-thyroid axis, and since the effect is most potent with central TRH administration, it would appear likely that TRH's analeptic actions are mediated by the CNS.

2. Other hypothalamo-adenohypophyseal polypeptides, amino acid fragments of TRH, TRH metabolites (e.g., deamidated TRH), classical neurotransmitters, and many psychopharmacologic agents have all been shown to be mainly ineffective (or their role is unclear) in altering the TRH analeptic effect. In contrast, only TRH and certain (perhaps properly spatially-oriented) structural analogues are effective in producing this effect. Their efficacy appears to be dissociated from their competitive binding affinities in pituitary TRH receptor preparations and their TSH release potencies in pituitary tissue preparations (Breese et al., 1975; Prange et al., 1975). It is most important to note that competitive radioreceptor TRH binding studies in pituitary tissues reveal highly specific saturable binding, a phenomenon found to be critical to *in vivo* biological potency—TSH release and PRL release (Burt and Snyder, 1975; Burt and Taylor, 1980; Grant et al., 1973; Vale et al., 1977). Therefore, an analogous relationship between the behavioral aspects of TRH antagonism of barbiturate-induced sleep and specific competitive radioreceptor TRH binding in CNS tissues could be proposed.

3. TRH and its effective analogues do not show a dose-response relationship for the analeptic effect after intraperitoneal (i.p.) administration (Breese et al., 1975; Prange et al., 1975). However, this mode of administration can be expected to render the peptide vulnerable to enzyme catabolism (Eskay et al., 1976). Also, as pointed out by Prange et al. (1974), and directly tested by Stumpf

and Sar (1973), only a small amount of parenterally administered TRH reaches the brain as compared with the amount that reaches the pituitary. Presumably TRH and its structural analogues must cross the blood–brain barrier in order to antagonize pentobarbital (Bissette et al., 1976; Prange et al., 1974, 1975). It could be proposed, however, that central TRH administrations might display dose-response relationships since problems of the parenteral route would be avoided.

4. (a) TRH-pentobarbital combinations show dose-related toxic and/or lethal effects (Breese et al., 1974b, 1975; Cohn et al., 1976; Crowley and Hydinger, 1976, 1977; Holaday et al., 1978; Prange et al., 1978b).

(b) In addition, as a result of a discrepancy between the biological activity constant of TRH (relative TSH release potency) empirically derived from *in vitro* secretion studies versus the binding affinity constant (K_A) found in pituitary receptor experiments (the former constant is tenfold lower than the latter), a "spare receptor" theory has been advanced (Grant et al., 1973; Vale et al., 1973; Vale and Rivier, 1975). Only a small percentage of receptors need be saturated (occupied) by TRH in order to produce a maximal biological response. Therefore, TRH's "secretory stimulation" curve is shifted to the left of its "binding" curve. Likewise, a "ceiling effect" could also be predicted for TRH's analeptic actions: only a small percentage of occupied central TRH receptors would be required for full analeptic actions. Beyond certain "limits," higher doses of TRH would no longer augment the analeptic action.

(c) It is also important to note that the overall dissociation of TRH away from its pituitary receptor does not follow simple first-order kinetics. The 50% dissociation rate determined by "infinite" dilution in the presence of excess unlabeled TRH is approximately three times more rapid than with "volumetric (no ligand)" dilution alone. In light of "the unusual kinetics of [TRH] binding to its receptor, its dissociation from the receptor, and the slightly different slopes in the competition curves," Vale and Rivier (1975) suggested the phenomenon of "negative cooperativity" as an alternate interpretation of the [^{3}H]-TRH competitive binding data. As De Meyts (1976) pointed out, "negative cooperativity" has several advantages over a "multiple class of [affinity] binding sites" type model: It requires no energy-dependent cell machinery, and only a single protein species undergoing conformational changes.

One might therefore expect that higher dose combinations of peptide-barbiturate would yield significant interaction effects and/or are nondose related as a function of either toxic interactions, or space receptor phenomena, or negative cooperativity phenomena.

5. Breese et al. (1975) found that peripherally administered TRH effectively interacted with barbiturate up to 30 minutes prior to i.p. pentobarbital administrations, but not at longer interinjection durations. Since the dissociation of TRH from its binding sites in the cerebral cortex has a half-life of about 38 minutes (Burt and Snyder, 1975), and since exogenous TRH is enzymatically destroyed in brain homogenates after 30 minutes at 37°C incubations (Winokur et al., 1977), exogenous central TRH (i.vt.) administrations would also be expected to decrease significantly after 30–40 minutes.

Several of these critical issues were directly tested in our laboratory (Hirsch, 1982). Male CF-1 mice, two months of age, were centrally (i.vt.) administered TRH pretreatments in conjunction with parenteral (i.p.) pentobarbital treatments (50 mg/kg). When TRH was administered at 1 minute before the barbiturate (1-minute interinjection duration, or IID), there was a dose-response relationship for the peptide analeptic effect. At a 10 µg/5 µl TRH dose, barbiturate narcosis was reduced by 41% from the saline baseline level; at a 20 µg/5 µl TRH dose, the narcosis was reduced by 60% from baseline. However, when TRH was administered at 45 minutes before the barbiturate (45-minute IID), the dose-response relationship was disrupted; that is, TRH's analeptic actions were attenuated toward baseline. The former findings would thus indicate, as proposed earlier, that central TRH injections are more effective than peripheral routes of administration due to: (a) an avoidance of the inherent problems of the latter route, and (b) the fact that the peptide mechanism is probably a central one. That TRH acts as a central analeptic rather than as a motor stimulant is borne out by Breese et al.'s (1974a) report that TRH pretreatments antagonize ethanol-induced narcosis in mice while amphetamines potentiate it. Also in their study, it was found that the peptide induced only mild increases in spontaneous locomotor activities of unanesthetized animals, whereas amphetamines markedly increased it. Additionally, Crowley and Hydinger (1976, 1977) reported that lower parenteral (i.m.) doses of TRH to normal monkeys has very little effect upon their motor activities, while higher doses reduce them, thus further dissociating the peptide's central analeptic effects from possibly altered motor activities.

The latter 45-minute IID results of our study support the findings cited earlier, which indicated that TRH was effective as an

analeptic up to a 30–40-minute IID. A subsequent pentobarbital
assay further indicated that in comparison with saline pretreatments, central peptide pretreatments did not alter regional brain
levels of the barbiturate (18.0–20.2 μg/g original tissue) at one hour
following pentobarbital administrations. It could therefore be
proposed that TRH does not influence hepatic metabolism of
barbiturates, a finding previously reported by Breese et al. (1975).
   When three-month-old male mice were tested under a factorial
paradigm utilizing different dose combinations of TRH-
pentobarbital, it was again found that the peptide was a potent
analeptic at both moderate (10 μg) and high (20 μg) TRH dose
pretreatments. However, the peptide did not display dose-response
relationships for this age group. In line with these latter results,
there were also dose-related toxic and lethal effects for TRH-
pentobarbital combinations: (a) Twenty-nine percent of the
animals died after receiving 20 μg TRH (i.vt.) plus 70 mg
pentobarbital/kg (i.p.); 9% died after saline plus 50 mg
pentobarbital/kg; 0% died after either 0 μg (saline), 10 μg, or
20 μg TRH plus saline (0 mg/kg, i.p.). (b) All animals receiving
peptide plus barbiturate displayed a distinct sequelae that might be
related to toxic and/or lethal drug interaction effects. This sequelae
has been described by a number of other investigators (Breese et
al., 1974b, 1975; Cohn et al., 1976; Crowley and Hydinger, 1976,
1977; Holaday et al., 1978; Prange et al., 1978b). The animals
appeared to be marginally asleep, although they displayed complete
loss of both righting reflexes and purposeful movements. The
animals additionally displayed frequent stereotypic scratching and
grooming, as well as shivering, shaking, tremors, and several
myoclonic-tonic convulsions.
   The fact that pentobarbital induced longer narcosis and greater
toxic effects in three-month-old mice than in two-month-olds, and
conversely, the fact that the peptide was a more effective analeptic
in the younger group, implicates an early critical stage in the
ontogenesis of the mouse responsivity to both of these pharmacologic agents. A second subsequent pentobarbital assay of
regional mouse brain tissues indicated that while central TRH
infusions per se again did not alter brain levels of barbiturate, there
were profound age-related differences in brain barbiturate levels at
1.5 hours after its parenteral (i.p.) administration. Thus it can be
proposed that there are early developmental changes in hepatic
barbiturate metabolism, a finding previously reported by other
workers (Kato et al., 1961; Stohs et al., 1980; Streicher and Garbus,
1955).

TRH DISTRIBUTION IN THE CNS

Brownstein et al. (1974) utilized a micropunch technique on frozen rat brain tissues to obtain discrete nuclei for identification of immunoreactive TRH via RIA. TRH was found in highest concentrations in hypothalamic regions. The median eminence had the highest TRH level (25% of total hypothalamic content) for this brain region, which was fourfold higher than for the ventromedial nucleus, the next highest area. High TRH concentrations were also found scattered among several other hypothalamic regions, in the following descending order: periventricular, dorsomedial, arcuate, and paraventricular nuclei. The preoptic area contained moderate TRH levels. The septal region also contained high TRH concentrations, especially in the lateral nucleus, followed by the dorsal nucleus. Thus endogenous TRH was localized predominantly within the area adjacent to ventricle III in the hypothalamic region and adjacent to the lateral ventricle in the septum. It is likely that TRH-barbiturate interactions are mediated within many of these hypothalamic, preoptic, and septal brain regions.

Indirect immunofluorescent microscopy has provided further evidence for TRH localization and extends earlier RIA data for the localization of TRH in the axon nerve terminal (Hökfelt et al., 1975); in addition, moderate to high TRH concentrations are found in both central (preoptic, septal, and brain stem motor nuclei) and peripheral (ventral horn of spinal cord) extrahypothalamic regions.

Youngblood et al. (1978) separated TRH-like substances from several regions of the rat brain by thin-layer chromatography (TLC). The immunoreactive (RIA) "elution profiles" obtained indicated that the hypothalamic and septal-preoptic regions might contain authentic TRH.

Spindel and Wurtman (1980) fractionated extracts from rat brain homogenate and via either TLC or high-pressure liquid chromatography (HPLC) isolated components from which TRH was identified immunoreactively by RIA. They identified specific immunoreactive TRH in many brain areas that had chromatographic characteristics that closely corresponded to synthetic TRH. This finding was validated by five different variations of their procedures. They reported finding authentic TRH in the frontal cortex, hypothalamus, septum, preoptic area, corpus striatum, and brain stem. Spindel and Wurtman suggest that Youngblood et al. may have failed to identify authentic TRH in other brain areas because of poor recoveries from multiple extracts as well as non-specific interfering compounds eluted, problems that they claim to have avoided.

Kubek and colleagues (1979) identified high levels of immuno-reactive TRH via RIA in human hypothalamic nuclei and adjacent regions. Highest TRH concentrations were found in the median eminence area, followed by the arcuate nucleus; intermediate concentrations were found in the hypothalamic paraventricular and periventricular nuclei; lowest concentrations were found in the mammillary complex as well as posterior, supraoptic, and anterior hypothalamic nuclei. While the human brain levels were lower than those reported for the rat brain (Brownstein et al., 1974), there was generally a close correspondence in regional brain TRH concentrations between the two species. Kubek et al. also demon-strated the complete stability of endogenous TRH in the rat brain. Incubations of hypothalamic and cerebral cortex tissue extracts at 4°C for 16 hours did not display altered TRH, nor did intact tissues incubated at 25°C for one hour.

TRH AS A NEUROMODULATOR

In addition to its classically characterized adenohypophyseal actions, an extraendocrine central neuromodulatory role has been postulated for this peptide based upon several findings: its wide-spread and extremely high concentrations (Brownstein et al., 1974; Hökfelt et al., 1975; Kubek et al., 1979; Leppäluoto et al., 1978; Spindel and Wurtman, 1980; Youngblood et al., 1978); its localization within axon nerve terminals (Hökfelt et al., 1975; Winokur et al., 1977); the observation that microiontophoretic applications can produce altered neuronal spike frequencies (Dyer and Dyball, 1974; Renaud and Martin, 1975; Renaud et al., 1975, 1976; Winokur and Beckman, 1978; Yarbrough, 1976, 1978; Yarbrough and Singh, 1978); its central binding distribution (Burt and Snyder, 1975; Burt and Taylor, 1980; Ogawa et al., 1981); the fact that TRH alters neurotransmitter release and turnover in the brain (Heal and Green, 1979; Jessel and Richards, 1977; Keller et al., 1974; Malthe-Sørenssen et al., 1978); the fact that it can also be released from brain-derived synaptosomes in transmitter-like fashion (Schaeffer et al., 1977; Warberg et al., 1977); and its profound pharmacologic actions upon behavior (Bissette et al., 1976; Breese et al., 1974a, 1974b, 1975; Cohn et al., 1976; Crowley and Hydinger, 1976, 1977; Ehrensing and Kastin, 1976;

Holaday et al., 1978; Kalivas and Horita, 1979, 1980; Kulig, 1975; Plotnikoff et al., 1972; Prange and Wilson, 1972; Prange et al., 1974, 1975, 1978a, 1978b; Wilson et al., 1973).

In order to further verify whether TRH actually does function as a central neurotransmitter-neuromodulator, it would thus seem critical to demonstrate that TRH and some of its structural analogues are capable of specific high-affinity saturable binding at central TRH receptor sites.

Specific Saturable Binding

Burt and Snyder (1975) utilized [^{3}H]-TRH radioreceptor binding studies to investigate specific TRH binding in the rat brain. They found high concentrations of high-affinity TRH binding sites distributed in the cerebral cortex, hypothalamus, hippocampus, and midbrain regions, a finding confirmed and extended in the monkey brain by Ogawa et al. (1981). The affinity constant (K_A; or dissociation constant, $K_D = 1/K_A$) values obtained for the cerebral cortex TRH binding sites were found to be similar to pituitary K_A values. Both types of tissues showed similar, yet distinct, recognition requirements for a number of TRH structural analogues. A later study by Burt and Taylor (1980), which improved on the earlier technique by utilization of [^{3}H-Me-His^2]-TRH in order to discriminate high- versus low-affinity [^{3}H]-TRH binding sites, indicated that the highest concentration of specific TRH sites in the sheep brain was located in the nucleus accumbens-septal area. This brain region was also found to have distinct structural recognition requirements as compared with anterior pituitary sites. Thus these findings lend strong support to the high specificity requirements expected for physiologically relevant TRH receptors in the CNS. Second, the results further indicate that brain versus adenohypophyseal binding site recognition for TRH and its structural analogues can be distinguished in a mode similar to reports by Breese et al. (1975) and Prange et al. (1975) that analeptic actions of TRH analogues could be dissociated from adenohypophyseal biological activities (TSH release).

NEUROCHEMICAL-NEUROANATOMICAL CONSIDERATIONS

A central cholinergic mechanism has been implicated in the TRH analeptic effect: Breese et al. (1975) found that centrally administered atropine and its methyl derivative, two specific muscarinic acetylcholine (ACH) receptor antagonists, blocked TRH antagonism of pentobarbital narcosis. Peripheral administrations of methyl atropine, on the other hand, failed to produce this effect. Phentolamine, an adrenergic antagonist, was also without effect in this paradigm. These findings agree with the inverse relationship observed between brain ACH content and neuronal activity levels during altered states of consciousness (i.e., sleep arousal) following pentobarbital and other anesthetics versus convulsant drug administrations (Elliott et al., 1950; Giarman and Pepeu, 1962; Phillis, 1968, 1970; Richter and Crossland, 1949; Simon and Kuhar, 1975; Tobias et al., 1946). It has been suggested that transmitter release and hence subsequent metabolic degradation are under direct regulation by neuronal impulse flow. Consequently, barbiturate-induced depressant influences upon neuronal activities abnormally attentuate ACH turnover and/or augment central reserve pools of transmitter (Atweh et al., 1975; Simon et al., 1976; Simon and Kuhar, 1975); central stimulatory influences like those of TRH are assumed to effect increased transmitter turnover and/or depletions of their pools (Malthe-Sørenssen et al., 1978).

Further support for a cholinergic mechanism is found in Yarbrough's (1976, 1978) and Yarbrough and Singh's (1978) reports that TRH applications can potentiate the excitatory actions of microiontophoretically applied ACH and carbamylcholine (carbachol) in the muscarinically identified somatosensory cortex of pentobarbital anesthetized rats.

A cholinergic component of the ascending reticular activating systems (ARAS), implicated in arousal, has been anatomically identified by experimental and histochemical specific cholinesterase-staining techniques (Lewis and Henderson, 1980; Shute and Lewis, 1963, 1967). The ARAS consists of dorsal and ventral cholinergic tegmental pathways of both mesencephalic reticular formation (MRF) and substantia nigra origins, respectively, which are then relayed to tectal, thalamic, and basal forebrain areas, and then further projected to the cerebral cortex and olfactory bulb. These pathways are closely related to the thalamic and extrathalamic portions of the ARAS. Classical experiments strongly implicate the ARAS in the mediation of altered states of consciousness during normal sleep–wakefulness as well as during stimulatory-inhibitory influences (Bradley, 1958; French and Magoun, 1952; Lindsley et al., 1950; Livingston, 1959; Moruzzi and Magoun, 1949). Both atropine and pentobarbital act within levels of this system (Bradley, 1958; Phillis, 1968). It is thus likely that TRH's antagonistic actions toward barbiturate narcosis are localized within various levels of this arousal system.

It is not clear, however, whether TRH-barbiturate interactions influence only the cholinergic components of this arousal system, or whether other noncholinergic transmitter components may also be involved in the analeptic effect since (a) noncholinergic corticopetal fibers of thalamic reticular origin are still capable of inducing cortical electroencephalogram (EEG) desynchronization responses following atropine administrations during reticular stimulations (Shute and Lewis, 1967); (b) monoamine-containing fibers can influence the cortical EEG (Fuxe, 1965); and (c) both TRH and barbiturates influence other transmitter systems of the brain, including norepinephrine, dopamine, serotonin, γ-aminobutyric acid, glutamic acid, and possibly glycine and histamine (Cott and Engel, 1977; Green and Grahame-Smith, 1974; Heal and Green, 1979; Huidobro-Toro et al., 1974; Jessel and Richards, 1977; Keller et al., 1974; Lotti et al., 1980; Plotnikoff et al., 1972; Renaud et al., 1976; Tabakoff et al., 1978; Waller and Richter, 1980; Winokur and Beckman, 1978).

On the other hand, Burt and Snyder (1975) and Burt and Taylor (1980) tested a large series of transmitters and related drugs and found that all agents tested—including carbachol, atropine, d-tubocurarine, and oxtremorine—lacked effective competitive displacement activities in [^{3}H]-TRH radioreceptor assays. It thus is likely that TRH's analeptic actions are not directly related to any other putative extra-TRH transmitter receptor actions. Hence TRH's analeptic effect may be directly related to only a specific TRH binding site-mediated action. Nonetheless, TRH binding sites might still be adjacent to or impinge upon other transmitter systems of the ARAS.

Additionally, it seems likely that the neuroanatomical focus of the analeptic effect must be further expanded. Green (1960) and Green and Arduini (1954) reported that pentobarbital narcosis is accompanied by neocortical EEG synchrony as well as asynchronous hippocampal discharges that interrupt the normal "theta" rhythm. It has been suggested that the "theta" rhythm represents hippocampal arousal since (a) the response occurs following sensory stimulation that also produces behavioral and cortical arousal; (b) the hippocampus receives direct connections from septal, entorhinal, and presubiculum regions of the limbic cortex; and (c) the hippocampus sends efferent fibers to the hypothalamus, the diffuse thalamic projection system, and the brain stem reticular formation (BSRF) (Green, 1960; Green and Arduini, 1954). Therefore, pentobarbital actions may also involve the hippocampus and other interconnected brain regions, which include the limbic forebrain and limbic brain stem. This viewpoint would agree with Ranson's

(1939) finding that lesions of the mammillary body and posterior hypothalamus—two main projection areas of the hippocampus—produce a profound somnolence, a finding further supported by Nauta's (1946) report that different regions of the hypothalamus are involved in the mediation of arousal-sleep states.

Green and Arduini (1954) propose that hippocampal activities can be subsumed under Papez's (1937) theory that the limbic rhinencephalon serves to integrate affective and visceral activities of higher levels of the CNS. Pentobarbital's anesthetic activities appear to involve brain regions within and innervated by the entire Papez limbic circuit. Pentobarbital markedly decreases neuronal activities in the cerebral cortex, hippocampus, and hypothalamus; septal stimulation significantly reverses these effects (Atweh et al., 1975; Simon et al., 1976; Simon and Kuhar, 1975). It is therefore important to note that both the analeptic actions and specific high-affinity binding sites of TRH have been localized within both forebrain and brain stem areas of the limbic circuit. Kalivas and Horita (1979, 1980) utilized a microinjection technique to administer TRH to discrete neuroanatomical sites in the rat following pentobarbital narcosis.

The septal region was found to be the most sensitive brain site for inducing TRH analeptic actions. Other highly sensitive brain sites include the nucleus accumbens, the medial thalamus, the interpenduncular nucleus, the medial preoptic area, the medial hypothalamus, the diencephalic-mesencephalic periventricular gray regions, and the locus ceruleus. Moderate sensitivities were also reported for the dorsal hippocampus, MRF, the substantia nigra, and the parafasicular nucleus. In this regard it is significant that Ogawa et al.'s (1981) [^{3}H]-TRH radioreceptor assay results indicated that the highest levels of specific high-affinity TRH binding sites of the monkey brain are localized within the limbic hippocampus and amygdala regions; the next highest levels are in the frontal cortex, interpeduncular nucleus, and periaqueductal gray matter of the midbrain. These radioreceptor findings agree with similar reports by Burt and Snyder (1975) and Burt and Taylor (1980). These latter two groups of investigators found that the nucleus accumbens has the highest concentration of TRH binding sites.

The Neuroanatomical Substrate of the TRH Analeptic Effect

Two direct tests were performed in our laboratory to determine the viability of considering central TRH receptors as the site of mediation for the analeptic effect (Hirsch, 1982).

1. Purified presynaptic and postsynaptic membranes of regional mouse brain tissue origin were prepared by the differential and density gradient centrifugation procedures of W. B. and S. G. Essman (1977) and E. J. and W. B. Essman (1980) respectively [as modified from Israel and Whittaker (1965) and Cotman et al. (1974) respectively]. Both De Robertis (1971) and Cotman and Taylor (1972) have independently characterized these purified synaptosomal membrane preparations as morphologically and physiologically functional neurotransmitter receptors. The barbiturate analogues phenobarbital, pentobarbital, and thiopental were tested as competitive inhibitors in the *in vitro* [^{3}H]-TRH radioreceptor assays. The results indicated that the limbic fore-brain region—which included the septal-hippocampal system and the hypothalamus—displayed the highest concentrations of both presynaptic and postsynaptic specific TRH high-affinity binding sites, as well as high degrees of competitive displacement by the barbiturate analogues. The 185.5–195.1 fmol/mg protein binding site concentrations observed for these receptors were values well within the ranges reported by Burt and Snyder (1975), Burt and Taylor (1980), and Ogawa et al. (1981) for this same brain region. Therefore, the fact that the barbiturate analogues inhibited [^{3}H]-TRH binding by as much as 45–96% strongly implicates the TRH binding sites of the limbic forebrain as the neuroanatomical substrate for the TRH analeptic effect.

2. These *in vitro* results are in line with the *in vivo* findings of Kalivas and Horita (1979, 1980). They are also in line with the results of the second direct study in our laboratory. Five micro-liters of 5 nM [^{3}H]-TRH were centrally administered *in vivo* into the right lateral ventricle of the mouse brain at 1 minute prior to either physiological (0.9%) saline or 50 mg pentobarbital/kg (i.p.) injections. At one-hour posttreatments, mice were killed, brains were rapidly removed over ice (0°C), coronal tissue sections were obtained, and discrete nuclei were dissected under a light microscope. The discrete nuclei were subsequently separated into soluble versus particulate fractions by centrifugation pro-cedures. Particulate fractions were then solubilized by Triton X-100. Finally, scintillation cocktail was added to all unknown, standard, and blank samples, and tritiation was read in a liquid scintillation counter. The results again indicated that the highest concentrations of total and particulate tritiated TRH ([^{3}H]-TRH plus saline group) were in the same limbic forebrain regions (septal-hippocampal system and hypothalamus), which were then subse-

quently displaced by barbiturate ([^{3}H]-TRH plus pentobarbital group).

It is important to note that the brain stem region was also found to contain a high concentration of specific presynaptic binding sites in the *in vitro* radioreceptor assay. These sites possessed a high affinity for both [^{3}H]-TRH and barbiturates (competitive displacement), data that fit in with the ARAS hypothesis cited earlier for TRH's analeptic effect. On the other hand, a [^{3}H]-TRH kinetic dissociation assay indicated that the brain stem TRH receptors display retention phenomena. This latter evidence would tend to preclude acceptance of the brain stem as a viable site for mediating the TRH analeptic effect. The *in vivo* radiochemical data further add to this disclaimer: While barbiturate administrations did not alter the low level of brain-stem particulate-bound tritiation from saline baseline levels, the drug did induce a 160% increase in soluble tritiation above baseline. Additionally, the cerebral cortex region was found to have the lowest concentration of specific postsynaptic TRH receptors— receptors that displayed the lowest TRH affinities. This CNS region displayed marked increases in [^{3}H]TRH in the *in vitro* barbiturate competitive displacement radioassays, in the [^{3}H]-TRH kinetic assays, and in the *in vivo* radiochemical assays. Thus the limbic forebrain region appears to be the only viable site for TRH-barbiturate interactions.

SUMMARY AND CONCLUSIONS

To summarize, this chapter has focused on the following areas of investigation related to TRH's CNS activities.

1. Chromatographic and immunocytochemical studies to localize endogenous TRH regionally within the CNS

2. Microiontophoretic experiments to identify generally functional active central TRH sites

3. Behavioral pharmacology studies to assess TRH-barbiturate dose-response relationships (main versus interaction effects), as well as the subsequent influences of altered interinjection durations and age upon these relationships

4. Biochemical assays to determine the effects of central TRH administrations and age factors upon regional brain levels of pentobarbital

5. *In vitro* competitive displacement [^{3}H]-TRH radioreceptor assays: (a) to identify the regional brain distribution of specific high-affinity TRH binding sites; and (b) to determine whether barbiturates act as competitive inhibitors at specific TRH binding sites

6. *In vivo* radiochemical assays to determine the regional brain distribution of [^{3}H]-TRH-pentobarbital sites of interaction

With specific regard to TRH's central analeptic actions, it can generally be concluded that:

1. TRH may sometimes display dose-response relationships.

2. These dose relationships seem to be functionally associated with temporal and ontogenetic characteristics of either specific central TRH receptors or nonspecific sites of peptide-barbiturate interactions.

3. The limbic forebrain region appears to be the neuroanatomical substrate for the peptide's analeptic effect.

4. TRH binding sites can be further discriminated as presynaptic versus postsynaptic, with regionally distinct peptide and barbiturate affinities and efficacies.

5. TRH might function as an extrapituitary central neuromodulator.

Clearly, the heuristic value of this research lies in a series of interrelated approaches (across the five previously cited levels) to TRH central neuromodulation and its antagonism of barbiturate-induced narcosis. From a pragmatic viewpoint, such data could suggest possible clinical approaches to the management of medical (anesthesia) and nonmedical (drug abuse) barbiturate overdoses.

REFERENCES

Atweh, S., Simon, J. R., and Kuhar, M. J. Utilization of sodium-dependent high affinity choline uptake *in vitro* as a measure of the activity of cholinergic neurons *in vivo*. *Life Sci.* 1975; 17:1535-1544.

Barbeau, A., Gonce, M., and Kastin, A. J. (1976): Neurologically active peptides. *In The Neuropeptides: Pharmacology Biochemistry and Behavior*, Vol. 5, suppl. 1, pp. 159-163.

Barker, J. L., Neale, J. H., Smith, T. G., Jr., and MacDonald, R. L. Opiate peptide modulation of amino acid responses suggests a novel form of neuronal communication. *Science* 1978; 199:1451-1453.

Bergland, R., Blume, H., Hamilton, A., Monica, P., and Paterson, R. Adrenocorticotropic hormone may be transported directly from the pituitary to the brain. *Science* 1980; 210:541-543.

Bissette, G., Nemeroff, C. B., Loosen, P. T., Prange, A. J., Jr., and Lipton, M. A. (1976): Comparison of the analeptic potency of TRH, ACTH

4-10, LHRH, and related peptides. *In The Neuropeptides: Pharmacology Biochemistry and Behavior,* Vol., 5, suppl. 1, pp. 135-138.

Bloom, F., Segal, D., Ling, N., and Guillemin, R. Endorphins: Profound behavioral effects in rats suggest new etiological factors in mental illness. *Science* 1976; 194:630-632.

Bowers, C. Y., Sievertsson, H., Chang, J., Stewart, J., Castensson, S., Bjorkman, S., Chang, K., and Folkers, K. (1976): TRH analog antagonists. *In* J. Robbins, L. E. Braverman, F. J. Ebling, and I. W. Henderson (Eds.), *Thyroid Research: Proceedings of the Seventh International Thyroid Conference—Boston, Massachusetts, June 9-13, 1975.* New York: American Elsevier Publishing Co., Inc.

Bradley, P. B. (1958): The central action of certain drugs in relation to the reticular formation of the brain. *In* H. H. Jasper, L. D. Proctor, R. S. Knighton, W. C. Noshay, and R. T. Costello (Eds.), *Reticular Formation of the Brain.* Boston: Little, Brown & Co.

Breese, G. R., Cott, J. M., Cooper, B. R., Prange, A. J., Jr., and Lipton, M. A. Antagonism of ethanol narcosis by thyrotropin releasing hormone. *Life Sci.* 1974; 14:1053-1063.

Breese, G. R., Cott, J. M., Cooper, B. R., Prange, A. J., Jr., Lipton, M. A., and Plotnikoff, N. P. Effects of thyrotropin-releasing hormone (TRH) on the actions of pentobarbital and other centrally acting drugs. *T. J. Pharmacol. Exper. Ther.* 1975; 193:11-22.

Breese, G. R., Cott, J. M., Cooper, B. R., Prange, A. J., Plotnikoff, N. P., and Lipton, M. A. Interaction of thyrotropin releasing hormone with various centrally-acting depressants. *Pharmacologist* 1974; 16:296. (abstract)

Browne, R. G., and Segal, D. S. Alterations in β-endorphin-induced locomotor activity in morphine-tolerant rats. *Neuropharmacology* 1980; 19: 619-621.

Brownstein, M. J. (1978): Are hypothalamic hormones central neuro-transmitters? *In* J. Hughes (Ed.), *Centrally Acting Peptides.* Baltimore: University Park Press.

Brownstein, J. J., Palkovits, M., Saavedra, J. M., Bassiri, R. M., and Utiger, R. D. Thyrotropin-releasing hormone in specific nuclei of rat brain. *Science* 1974, 185:267-269.

Burt, D. R., and Snyder, S. H. Thyrotropin releasing hormone (TRH): Apparent receptor binding in rat brain membranes. *Brain Res.* 1975; 93:309-328.

Burt, D. R., and Taylor, R. L. Binding sites for thyrotropin-releasing hormone in sheep nucleus accumbens resemble pituitary receptors. *Endocrinology* 1980; 106:1416-1423.

Chang, J., Fong, B. T. W., Pert, A., and Pert, C. B. Opiate receptor affinities and behavioral effects of enkephalin: Structure-activity relationships of ten synthetic peptide analogues. *Life Sci.* 1976; 18:1473-1482.

Cohn, M. L., Cohn, M., Krzysik, B. A., and Taylor, F. H. (1976): Regulation of behavioral events by thyrotropin releasing factor and cyclic AMP. *In The Neuropeptides Pharmacology Biochemistry and Behavior,* Vol. 5, suppl. 1, pp. 129-133.

Cooper, J. R., Bloom, F. E., and Roth, R. H. (1978): *The Biochemical Basis of Neuropharmacology.* New York: Oxford University Press.

Cotman, C. W., and Taylor, D. Isolation and structural studies on synaptic complexes from rat brain. *J. Cell Biol.* 1972; 55:696-711.

Cotman, C. W., Banker, G., Churchill, L., and Taylor, D. Isolation of post-synaptic densities from rat brain. *J. Cell Biol.* 1974; 63:441-455.

Cott, J., and Engel, J. Antagonism of the analeptic activity of thyrotropin-releasing hormone (TRH) by agents which enhance GABA transmission. *Psychopharmacology* 1977; 52:145-149.

Creese, I., and Snyder, S. H. Receptor binding and pharmacological activity of opiates in the guinea-pig intestine. *J. Pharmacol. Exper. Ther.* 1975; 194:205-219.

Crowley, T. J., and Hydinger, M. (1976): MIF, TRH, and simian social and motor behavior. *In The Neuropeptides: Pharmacology Biochemistry and Behavior*, Vol. 5, suppl. 1, pp. 79-87.

Crowley, T. J., and Hydinger, M. Comparison of thyrotropin-releasing hormone with melanocyte-stimulating-hormone-release-inhibiting factor as pentobarbital antagonists in monkeys. *Psychopharmacology* 1977; 53:205-206.

De Meyts, P. (1976): The negative cooperativity of insulin receptors: A model for the regulation of hormone recognition by target cells. *In Viruses, Antigens and Antibodies, Polypeptide Hormones, and Small Molecules.* New York: Raven Press.

De Robertis, E. Ultrastructure and cytochemistry of the synapse: Isolation and nature of receptors in the central nervous system. *Adv. Cyto-pharmacology* 1971; 1:291-300.

De Wied, D. (1974): Pituitary adrenal system hormones and behaviour. *In* F. O. Schmitt and F. G. Worden (Eds.), *The Neurosciences: Third Study Program.* Cambridge, Mass.: MIT Press.

De Wied, D. (1978): Behavioural effects of neuropeptides related to β-LPH. *In* J. Hughes (Ed.), *Centrally Acting Peptides.* Baltimore: University Park Press.

Dyer, R. G., and Dyball, R. E. J. Evidence for a direct effect of LRF and TRF on single unit activity in the rostral hypothalamus. *Nature* 1974; 252:486-488.

Ehrensing, R. H., and Kastin, A. J. (1976): Clinical investigations for emotional effects of neuropeptide hormones. *In The Neuropeptides: Pharmacology Biochemistry and Behavior*, Vol. 5, suppl. 1, pp. 89-93.

Elliott, K. A. C., Swank, R. L., and Henderson, N. Effects of anesthetics and convulsants on acetylcholine content of the brain. *Am. J. Physiol.* 1950; 162:469-474.

Eskay, R. L., Oliver, C., Warberg, J., and Porter, J. C. Inhibition of degradation and measurement of immuno-reactive thyrotropin-releasing hormone in rat blood plasma. *Endocrinology* 1976; 98:269-277.

Essman, E. J., and Essman, W. B. Synaptosomal GABA uptake and receptor binding: Effects of a convulsion. *Brain Res. Bull.* 1980; 5(suppl. 2): 209-211.

Essman, W. B., and Essman, S. G. (1977): Amine regulation of protein synthesis in retrograde amnesia. *In* J. M. R. Delgado and F. DeFeudis (Eds.), *Behavioral Neurochemistry.* New York: Spectrum Publishing.

Ferris, S. H., Sathananthan, G., Gershon, S., Clark, C., and Moshinsky, J. (1976): Cognitive effects of ACTH 4-10 in the elderly. *In The Neuropeptides: Pharmacology Biochemistry and Behavior*, Vol. 5, suppl. 1, pp. 73-78.

Flood, J. F., Jarvik, M. E., Bennett, E. L., and Orme, A. E. (1976): Effects of ACTH peptide fragments on memory formation. *In The Neuro-*

peptides: Pharmacology Biochemistry and Behavior, Vol. 5, suppl. 1, pp. 41-51.

French, J. D., and Magoun, H. W. Effects of chronic lesions in central cephalic brain stem of monkeys. *Arch. Neurol. Psychiat.* 1952; 68: 591-604.

Fuxe, K. The distribution of monoamine terminals in the central nervous system. *Acta Physiol. Scand.* 1965; 64(suppl. 247):37-120.

Giarman, N. J., and Pepeu, G. Drug-induced changes in brain acetylcholine. *Br. J. of Pharmacol. Chemother.* 1962; 19:226-234.

Gintzler, A. R. Endorphin-mediated increases in pain threshold during pregnancy. *Science* 1980; 210:193-195.

Gold, P. W., Goodwin, F. K., Post, R. M., and Robertson, G. L. Vasopressin function in depression and mania. *Psychopharmacol. Bull.* 1981; 17: 7-9.

Goldstein, A. Opioid peptides (endorphins) in pituitary and brain. *Science* 1976; 193:1081-1086.

Goldstein, A., Tachibana, S., Lowney, L. I., Hunkapiller, M., and Hood, L. Dynorphin—(1-13), an extraordinarily potent opioid peptide. *Proc. Nat. Acad. Sci. U.S.A.* 1979; 76:6666-6670.

Grant, G., Vale, W., and Guillemin, R. Characteristics of the pituitary binding sites for thyrotropin-releasing factor. *Endocrinology* 1973; 92:1629-1633.

Green, A. R., and Grahame-Smith, D. G. TRH potentiates behavioural changes following increased brain 5-hydroxytryptamine accumulation in rats. *Nature* 1974; 251:524-526.

Green, J. D. (1960): The hippocampus. *In* J. Field, H. W. Magoun, and V. E. Hall (Eds.), *Handbook of Physiology*, Vol. 2, *Neurophysiology*. Washington, D.C.: American Physiological Society.

Green, J. D., and Arduini, A. A. Hippocampal electrical activity in arousal. *J. Neurophys.* 1954; 17:543-557.

Guillemin, R. Peptides in the brain: The new endocrinology of the neuron. *Science* 1978; 202:390-402.

Guillemin, R., Ling, N., and Burgus, R. (1976): Endorphines, peptides, d'origine hypothalamique et neurohypophysaire à activité morphinomimétique. Isolement et structure moléculaire de l' α-endorphine. *Comptes Rendus Hebdomadaires des séances de l' Academié des Sciences* 282(série D):783-785.

Haigler, H. J., and Spring, D. D. A comparison of the analgesic and behavioral effects of [D-Ala^2] metenkephalinamide and morphine in the mesencephalic reticular formation of rats. *Life Sci.* 1978; 23: 1229-1239.

Harris, G. W., Reed, M., and Fawcett, C. P. Hypothalamic releasing factors and the control of anterior pituitary function. *Br. Med. Bull.* 1966; 22:266-272.

Heal, D. J., and Green, A. R. Administration of thyrotropin releasing hormone (TRH) to rats releases dopamine in n. accumbens but not n. caudatus. *Neuropharmacology* 1979; 18:23-31.

Hirsch, M. D. Thyrotropin releasing hormone modulation of barbiturate anesthesia. *The Soc. for Neuroscience* 1982; 8(1):286. (abstract)

Ho, W. K. K., Wen, H. L., and Ling, N. Beta-endorphine-like immunoactivity in the plasma of heroin addicts and normal subjects. *Neuropharmacology* 1980; 19:117-120.

56	*Hirsch*

Hökfelt, T., Fuxe, K., Johansson, O., Jeffcoate, S., and White, N. Distribution of thyrotropin-releasing hormone (TRH) in the central nervous system as revealed with immunohistochemistry. *Eur. J. Pharmacol.* 1975; 34:389-392.

Holaday, J. W., Tseng, L.-F., Loh, H. H., and Li, C. H. Thyrotropin releasing hormone antagonizes β endorphin hypothermia and catalepsy. *Life Sci.* 1978; 22:1537-1544.

Hollister, L. E. (1973): *Clinical Use of Psychotherapeutic Drugs* (3rd printing). Springfield, Charles C Thomas.

Hollister, L. E., Kanter, S. L., and Clyde, D. J. Studies of prolonged-action medication. III. Pentobarbital sodium in prolonged-action form compared with conventional capsules: Serum levels of drugs and clinical effects following acute doses. *Clin. Pharmacol. Ther.* 1963; 4:612-618.

Hughes, J. Isolation of an endogenous compound from the brain with pharmacological properties similar to morphine. *Brain Res.* 1975; 88:295-308.

Hughes, J. (Ed.) (1978)· *Centrally Acting Peptides.* Baltimore: University Park Press.

Hughes, J., Smith, T W., Kosterlitz, H. W., Fothergill, L. A., Morgan, B. A., and Morris, H. R. Identification of two related pentapeptides from the brain with potent opiate agonist activity. *Nature* 1975; 258:577-579.

Huidobro-Toro, J. P., Scotti de Carolis, A., and Longo, V. G. Action of two hypothalamic factors (TRH, MIF) and of angiotensin II on the behavioral effects of L-Dopa and 5-hydroxytryptophan in mice. *Pharmacol. Biochem. Behav.* 1974; 2:105-109.

Israël, M., and Whittaker, V. P. The isolation of mossy fibre endings from the granular layer of the cerebellar cortex. *Experientia* 1965; 21: 325-326.

Jacquet, Y. F., Klee. W. A., and Smyth, D. G. β-endorphin: Modulation of acute tolerance and antagonism by endogeneous brain systems. *Brain Res.* 1978; 156:396-401.

Jacquet, Y. F., and Marks, N. The C-fragment of β-lipotropin: An endogenous neuroleptic or antipsychotogen? *Science* 1976; 194:632-635.

Jessell, T. M., and Richards, C. D. Barbiturate potentiation of hippocampal i.p.s.p.s. is not mediated by blockage of GABA uptake. *J. Physiol.* 1977; 269:42P-44P (abstract)

Kalivas, P. W., and Horita, A. Thyrotropin-releasing hormone: Central site of action in antagonism of pentobarbital narcosis. *Nature* 1979; 278:461-463.

Kalivas, P. W., and Horita, A. Thyrotropin-releasing hormone: Neurogenesis of actions in the pentobarbital narcotized rat. *J. Pharmacol. Exper. Ther.* 1980; 212:203-210.

Kato, R., Chiesara, E., and Frontino, G. Induced increase of meprobamate metabolism in rats pretreated with phenobarbital or phenaglycodol in relation to age. *Experientia* 1961; 17:520-521.

Katz, R. J. Behavioral effects of dynorphine—A novel opioid neuropeptide. *Neuropharmacology* 1980; 19:801-803.

Keller, H. H., Bartholini, G., and Pletscher, A. Enhancement of cerebral noradrenaline turnover by thyrotropin-releasing hormone. *Nature* 1974; 248 528-529.

Kosterlitz, H. W., and Waterfield, A. A. *In vitro* models in the study of structure-activity relationships of narcotic analgesics. *Ann. Rev. Pharmacol.* 1975; 15:29-47

Kubek, M., Wilber, J. F., and George, J. M. The distribution and concentration of thyrotropin-releasing hormone in discrete human hypothalamic nuclei. *Endocrinology* 1979; 105:537–540.

Kulig, B. M. The effects of thyrotropin-releasing hormone on the behaviour of rats pretreated with α-methyltyrosine. *Neuropharmacology* 1975; 14:489–492.

Labrie, F., Barden, N., Poirier, G., and De Lean, A. Binding of thyrotropin-releasing hormone to plasma membranes of bovine anterior pituitary gland. *Proc. Nat. Acad. Sci.* 1972; 69(1):283–287.

Labrie, F., De Lean, A., Lagrace, L., Drouin, J., Ferland, L., Beaulieu, M., and Morin, O. (1978): Interactions of TRH, LH-RH, and somatostatin in the anterior pituitary gland. *In* L. Birnbaumer and B. W. O'Mallery (Eds.), *Receptors and Hormone Action.* New York: Academic Press.

Lazarus, L. H., Ling, N., and Guillemin, R. β-lipotropin as a prohormone for the morphinomimetic peptides endorphins and enkephalins. *Proc. Nat. Acad. Sci., U.S.A.* 1976; 73:2156–2159.

Leppäluoto, J., Koivusalo, F., and Kraama, R. Thyrotropin-releasing factor: Distribution in neural and gastro-intestinal tissues. *Acta Physiol. Scand.* 1978; 104:175–179.

Lewis, P. R., and Henderson, Z. Tracing putative cholinergic pathways by a dual cytochemical technique. *Brain Res.* 1980; 196:489–493.

Lewis, R. V., Stern, A. S., Kimura, S., Rossier, J., Brink, L., Gerber, L. D., Stein, S., and Udenfriend, S. (1980): Opioid peptides and precursors in the adrenal medulla. *In* E. Costa and M. Trabucchi (Eds.), *In Neural Peptides and Neuronal Communication, Advances in Biochemical Psychopharmacology, Vol. 22.* New York: Raven Press, pp. 167–179.

Lindsley, D. B., Schreiner, L. H., Knowles, W. B., and Magoun, H. W. Behavioral and EEG changes following chronic brain stem lesions in the cat. *Electroencephal. Clin. Neurophys.* 1950; 2:483–498.

Livingston, R. B. (1959): Central control of receptors and sensory transmission systems. *In* J. Field, H. W. Magoun, and V. E. Hall (Eds.), *Handbook of Physiology, Vol. 1, Neurophysiology.* Baltimore: Williams & Wilkins.

Lotti, V. J., Yarbrough, G. G., and Clineschmidt, B. V. Investigations on the interaction of thyrotropin-releasing hormone (TRH) and MK-771 with central noradrenergic mechanisms. *Psychopharmacology* 1980; 70:145–148.

Lybeck, H., Leppäluoto, J., Virkkunen, P., Schafer, D., Carlsson, L., and Mulder, J. Suppression of TRH-mediated thyroidal release of ^{131}I by a synthetic analog. *Neuroendocrinology (Short Commun.)* 1973; 12:366–370.

Malthe-Sørenssen, D., Wood, P. L., Cheney, D. L., and Costa, E. Modulation of the turnover rate of acetylcholine in rat brain by intraventricular injections of thyrotropin-releasing hormone, somatostatin, neurotensin and angiotension II. *J. Neurochemistry* 1978; 31:685–691.

Martin, J. B., Renaud, L. P., and Brazeau, P. Hypothalamic peptides: New evidence for "peptidergic" pathways in the C.N.S. *Lancet* 1975; 2:393–395.

Miller, L. J., Harris, L. C., van Riezen, H., and Kastin, A. J. (1976): Neuroheptapeptide influence on attention and memory in man. *In The Neuropeptides Pharmacology Biochemistry and Behavior, Vol. 5, suppl. 1, pp. 17–21.*

Mortimer, C. H., McNeilly, A. S., Fisher, R. A., Murray, M. A. F., and Besser,
  G. M. Gonadotrophin-releasing hormone therapy in hypogonadal males
  with hypothalamic or pituitary dysfunction. *Br. Med. J.* 1974; 4:617-
  621.
Moruzzi, G., and Magoun, H. W. Brain stem reticular formation and activation
  of the EEG. *Electroenceph. Clin. Neurophys.* 1949; 1:455-473.
Nauta, W. J. H. Hypothalamic regulation of sleep in rats. An experimental
  study. *J. Neurophys.* 1946; 9:285-316.
Ogawa, N., Yamawaki, Y., Kuroda, H., Ofuji, T., Itoga, E., and Kito, S.
  Discrete regional distributions of thyrotropin releasing hormone (TRH)
  receptor binding in monkey central nervous system. *Brain Res.*
  1981; 205:169-174.
Papez, J. W. A proposed mechanism of emotion. *Arch. Neurol. Psychiatry*
  1937; 38:725-744.
Pearse, A. G. E. (1978): Diffuse neuroendocrine system: Peptides common
  to brain and intestine and their relationship to the APUD concept. *In*
  J. Hughes (Ed.), *Centrally Acting Peptides.* Baltimore: University Park
  Press.
Pert, A., Simantov, R., and Snyder, S. H. A morphine-like factor in
  mammalian brain: Analgesic activity in rats. *Brain Res.* 1977; 136:
  523-533.
Phillis, J. W. Acetylcholine release from the cerebral cortex: Its role in
  cortical arousal. *Brain Res.* 1968; 7:378-389.
Phillis, J. W. (1970): *The Pharmacology of Synapses.* Oxford: Pergamon
  Press.
Plotnikoff, N. P., Prange, A. J., Jr., Breese, G. R., Anderson, M. S., and
  Wilson, I. C. Thyrotropin releasing hormone: Enhancement of dopa
  activity by a hypothalamic hormone. *Science* 1972; 178:417-418.
Poirier, G., Labrie, F., Barden, N., and Lemaire, S. Thyrotropin-releasing
  hormone receptor: Its partial purification from bovine anterior pituitary
  gland and its close association with adenyl cyclase. *FEBS Lett.* 1972;
  20(3):283-286.
Pollard, H., Llorens-Cortes, C., and Schwartz, J. C. Enkephalin receptors on
  dopaminergic neurons in rat striatum. *Nature* 1977; 268:745-747.
Pomeranz, B. Brain's opiates at work in acupuncture? *New Scientist* 1977;
  73:12-13.
Prange, A. J., Jr., Breese, G. R., Cott, J. M., Martin, B. R., Cooper, B. R.,
  Wilson, I. C., and Plotnikoff, N. P. Thyrotropin releasing hormone:
  Antagonism of pentobarbital in rodents. *Life Sci.* 1974; 14:447-455.
Prange, A. J., Jr., Breese, G. R., Jahnke, G. D., Martin, B. R., Cooper, B. R.,
  Cott, J. M., Wilson, I. C., Alltop, L. B., Lipton, M. A., Bissette, G.,
  Nemeroff, C. B., and Loosen, P. T. Modification of pentobarbital
  effects by natural and synthetic polypeptides: Dissociation of brain
  and pituitary effects. *Life Sci.* 1975; 16:1907-1914.
Prange, A. J., Jr., Nemeroff, C. B., Lipton, M. A., Breese, G. R., and Wilson,
  I. C. (1978a): Peptides and the central nervous system. *In* L. L.
  Iversen, S. D. Iversen, and S. H. Snyder (Eds.), *Handbook of Psycho-
  pharmacology Biology of Mood and Antianxiety Drugs.* New York:
  Plenum Press.
Prange, A. J., Jr., Nemeroff, C. B., and Loosen, P. T. (1978b): Behavioral
  effects of hypothalamic peptides. *In* J. Hughes (Ed.), *Centrally Acting
  Peptides.* Baltimore: University Park Press.

Prange, A. J., Jr., and Wilson, I. C. Thyrotropin releasing hormone (TRH) for the immediate relief of depression: A preliminary report. *Psychopharmacologia* 1972; 26(suppl.):82. (abstract)

Ranson, S. W. Somnolence caused by hypothalamic lesions in the monkey. *Arch. Neurol. Psychiat.* 1939; 41:1-23.

Rees, H. D., Verhoef, J., Witter, A., Gispen, W. H., and De Wied, D. Autoradiographic studies with a behaviorally potent ^{3}H-ACTH$_{4-9}$ analog in the brain after intraventricular injection in rats. *Brain Res. Bull.* 1980; 5:509-514.

Renaud, L. P., and Martin, J. B. Thyrotropin releasing hormone (TRH): Depressant action on central neuronal activity. *Brain Res.* 1975; 86:150-154.

Renaud, L. P., Martin, J. B., and Brazeau, P. Depressant action of TRH, LH-RH and somatostatin on activity of central neurones. *Nature* 1975; 255:233-235.

Renaud, L. P., Martin, J. B., and Brazeau, P. (1976): Hypothalamic releasing factors: Physiological evidence for a regulatory action on central neurons and pathways for their distribution in brain. *In The Neuropeptides: Pharmacology Biochemistry and Behavior,* Vol. 5, suppl. 1, pp. 171-178.

Richter, D., and Crossland, J. Variation in acetylcholine content of the brain with physiological state. *Am. J. Physiol.* 1949; 159:247-255.

Rigter, H. Attenuation of amnesia in rats by systematically administered enkephalins. *Science* 1978; 200:83-85.

Rigter, H., Janssens-Elbertse, R., and van Riezen, H. (1976): Reversal of amnesia by an orally active ACTH 4-9 analog (Org 2766). *In The Neuropeptides: Pharmacology Biochemistry and Behavior,* Vol. 5, suppl. 1, pp. 53-58.

Roubicek, J., Krebs, E., and Poeldinger, W. Classification of endorphins/ enkephalins in brain physiology and pathology (based on EEG and clinical study of synthetically-modified methionine-enkephalin). *Progr. Neuropsychopharmacol.* 1980; 4:507-518.

Sandman, C. A., Miller, L. H., and Kastin, A. J. (1976): Proceedings of the bicentennial neuropeptide conference. *In The Neuropeptides: Pharmacology Biochemistry and Behavior,* Vol. 5, suppl. 1, p. 1.

Schaeffer, J. M., Axelrod, J., and Brownstein, M. J. Regional differences in dopamine-mediated release of TRH-like material from synaptosomes. *Brain Res.* 1977; 138:571-574.

Shute, C. C. D., and Lewis, P. R. Cholinesterase containing systems of the brain of the rat. *Nature* 1963; 199:1160-1164.

Shute, C. C. D., and Lewis, P. R. The ascending cholinergic reticular system: Neocortical, olfactory and subcortical projections. *Brain* 1967; 90:467-520.

Sievertsson, H., Castensson, S., Andersson, K., Björkman, S., and Bowers, C. Y. Thyrotropin and prolactin inhibitory studies by compounds related to the thyrotropin releasing hormone. *Biochem. Biophys. Res. Commun.* 1975; 66(4):1401-1407.

Simantov, R., and Snyder, S. H. Morphine-like peptides in mammalian brain: Isolation, structure elucidation and interactions with the opiate receptor. *Proc. Nat. Acad. Sci., U.S.A.* 1976; 73:2515-2519.

Simantov, R., and Snyder, S. H. Opiate receptor binding in the pituitary gland. *Brain Res.* 1977; 124:178-184.

Simon, J. R., and Kuhar, M. J. Impulse-flow regulation of high affinity choline uptake in brain cholinergic nerve terminals. *Nature* 1975; 255:162-163.

Simon, J. R., Atweh, S., and Kuhar, M. J. Sodium-dependent high affinity choline uptake: A regulatory step in the synthesis of acetylcholine. *J. Neurochemistry* 1976; 26:909-922.

Snyder, S. H., Uhl, G. R., and Kuhar, M. J. (1978): Comparative features of enkephalin and neurotensin in the mammalian central nervous system. *In* J. Hughes (Ed.), *Centrally Acting Peptides.* Baltimore: University Park Press.

Spindel, E., and Wurtman, R. J. TRH immunoreactivity in rat brain regions, spinal cord and pancreas: Validation by high-pressure liquid chromotography and thin-layer chromatography. *Brain Res.* 1980; 201:279-288.

Stohs, S. J., Al-Turk, W. A., and Hassing, J. M. Altered drug metabolism in hepatic and extrahepatic tissues in mice as a function of age. *Age* 1980; 3:88-92.

Streicher, E., and Garbus, J. The effect of age and sex on the duration of hexobarbital anesthesia in rats. *J. Gerontology* 1955; 10:441-444.

Stumpf, W. E., and Sar, M. ^{3}H-TRH and ^{3}H-proline radioactivity localization in pituitary and hypothalamus. *Fed. Proc.* 1973; 32(1):211. (abstract)

Swank, R. L., and Watson, C. W. Effects of barbiturates and anesthesia on spontaneous electrical activity of dog brain. *J. Neurophysiology* 1949; 12:137-148.

Tabakoff, B., Yanai, J., and Ritzmann, R. F. Brain noradrenergic systems as a prerequisite for developing tolerance to barbiturates. *Science* 1978; 200:449-451.

Tobias, J. M., Lipton, M. A., and Lepinat, A. A. Effect of anesthetics and convulsants on brain acetylcholine content. *Soc. Exp. Biol. Med.* 1946; 61:51-54.

Urban, I., and DeWied, D. Changes in excitability of the theta activity generating substrate by AHTH 4-10 in the rat. *Exp. Brain Res.* 1976; 24:325-334.

Vale, W., and Rivier, C. (1975): Hypothalamic hypophysiotropic hormones. *In* L. L. Iversen, S. D. Iversen, and S. H. Snyder (Eds.), *Handbook of Psychopharmacology,* Vol. 5. New York: Plenum Press.

Vale, W., Grant, G., and Guillemin, R. (1973): Chemistry of the hypothalamic releasing factors—Studies on structure-function relationships. *In* W. F. Ganong and L. Martini (Eds.), *Frontiers in Neuroendocrinology, 1973.* New York: Oxford University Press.

Vale, W., Rivier, C., and Brown, M. Regulatory peptides of the hypothalamus. *Ann. Rev. Physiol* 1977; 39:473-527.

Vale, W., Rivier, J., and Burgus, R. Synthetic TRF (thyrotropin releasing factor) analogues II. pGlu-N^{31} ^{m}Me-His-Pro-NH$_2$: A synthetic analogue with specific activity greater than that of TRF. *Endocrinology* 1971; 89:1485-1488.

Valzelli, L. (1973): W. B. Essman (Ed.), *Psychopharmacology.* New York: Spectrum Publishing.

Van Ree, J. M., and Otte, A. P. Effects of (Des-Try^1)-γ-endorphin and α-endorphin as compared to haloperidol and amphetamine on nucleus accumbens self-stimulation. *Neuropharmacology* 1980; 19:429-434.

Van Riezen, H., Rigter, H., and DeWied, D. Possible significance of ACTH fragments for human mental performance. *Behavioral Biol.* 1977; 20:311-324.

Waller, M. B., and Richter, J. A. Effects of pentobarbital and Ca^{2+} on the resting and K^+-stimulated release of several endogenous neurotransmitters from rat midbrain slices. *Biochemical Pharmacol.* 1980; 29: 2189-2198.

Warberg, J., Eskay, R. L., Barnea, A., Reynolds, R. C., and Porter, J. C. Release of luteinizing hormone releasing hormone and thyrotropin releasing hormone from a synaptosome-enriched fraction of hypothalamic homogenates. *Endocrinology* 1977; 100:814-825.

Wilson, I., Lara, P. P., and Prange, A. J., Jr. Thyrotropin-releasing hormone in schizophrenia. *Lancet* 1973; 819:43-44.

Wimersma Greidanus, Tj. B. van, and DeWied, D. (1976): Dorsal hippocampus: A site of action of neuropeptides on avoidance behavior? *In The Neuropeptides: Pharmacology Biochemistry and Behavior*, Vol. 5, suppl. 1, pp. 29-33.

Winokur, A., and Beckman, A. L. Effects of thyrotropin releasing hormone, norepinephrine and acetylcholine on the activity of neurons in hypothalamus, septum and cerebral cortex of the rat. *Brain Res.* 1978; 150:205-209.

Winokur, A., Davis, R., and Utiger, R. D. Subcellular distribution of thyrotropin-releasing hormone (TRH) in rat brain and hypothalamus. *Brain Res.* 1977; 120:423-434.

Yarbrough, G. G. TRH potentiates excitatory actions of acetylcholine on cerebral cortical neurons. *Nature* 1976; 263:523-524.

Yarbrough, G. G. Studies on the neuropharmacology of thyrotropin releasing hormone (TRH) and a new TRH analog. *Eur. J. Pharmacol.* 1978; 48 19-27.

Yarbrough, G. G., and Singh, D. K. Intravenous thyrotropin releasing hormone (TRH) enhances the excitatory actions of acetylcholine (ACH) on rat cortical neurons. *Experientia* 1978; 34:390.

Youngblood, W. W., Lipton, M. A., and Kizer, J. S. TRH-like immunoreactivity in urine, serum and extrahypothalamic brain: Non-identity with synthetic pyroglu-hist-pro-NH_2 (TRH). *Brain Res.* 1978; 151:99-116.

3

Diagnostic and Therapeutic Applications of Gastrointestinal Hormones

PREM MISRA
and
SELIM BARUH

The gastrointestinal hormones secretin and gastrin were discovered in 1902 and 1905 respectively. For many years it was taught that gastrin controlled gastric acid secretion, secretin controlled pancreatic bicarbonate, and cholecystokinin-pancreozymin controlled the contraction of the gallbladder and the enzyme output of the pancreas. Because of the development of such techniques as ion exchange chromatography, gel chromatography, affinity chromatography, radioimmunoassay, and isoelectric focusing, the decade of the 1970s led to a spectacular improvement in the isolation and chemical purification of many gut peptides.

Because the gut endocrine system is diffuse and not glandular or discrete, techniques of classical endocrinology, such as extirpation, often are not applicable, and the results of deficiency states therefore can not be studied easily. In addition, control of gut peptides is not always endocrine but neurocrine, and paracrine control is also involved. Furthermore, many gut hormones are common to brain and gut. Because of these considerations, much of the clinically useful knowledge about gut peptides is limited to neoplasms of the GI tract and pancreas, which cause states of overproduction of one or more of the gastrointestinal hormones.

Despite the marked increase in knowledge regarding gut hormones since the introduction of the Wiesbaden classification (1969) of endocrine cell types in the gut and its modification in Lausanne (1977), there is still no general agreement concerning the nomenclature for the different gut hormone-producing cells. Earlier nomenclature was based purely on histology; more recently, cells are being described according to the peptide they produce, in relation to neurotensin.

The following discussion deals in large part with the recognition, diagnosis, and treatment of syndromes of overproduction of gut hormones, but also briefly outlines our limited knowledge of the role of "eupeptides" or "gut peptides" in other disease states. The circumstances in which a clinician should request a radioimmunoassay or other determination of gut hormones are described. Although antibodies against islet cells have been described, techniques to recognize antibodies against the endocrine cells of the gut are not yet available.

Presently recognized tumor syndromes include those with secretion of gastrin, insulin, glucagon, pancreatic polypeptide, somatostatin, and vasoactive intestinal polypeptide, and of course the carcinoid syndrome. Patients with peptic ulcer disease, bullous skin rash, hypoglycemia, or watery diarrhea of unknown cause, or patients with tumors of the pancreas or small bowel or diabetes mellitus associated with one or more of the above features, should have the appropriate assay for either gastrin, insulin, glucagon, pancreatic polypeptide, somatostatin, or vasoactive intestinal polypeptide (VIP) performed.

ZOLLINGER-ELLISON SYNDROME

In 1955 Robert M. Zollinger and Edwin H. Ellison, from Ohio State University, described patients with the triad of gastric hydrochloric acid hypersecretion with fulminant ulcer diathesis, rapidly recurring despite adequate therapy, and non-B islet cell tumors of the pancreas. Gregory and Tracy (1964) showed that the pancreatic tumor produces gastrin. Early assays for gastrin were bioassays (Lai, 1964; Lambling et al., 1965). The advent of radioimmunoassays for gastrin (Hansky and Cain, 1969; McGuigan and Trudeau, 1970; Yalow and Berson, 1970; Stadil and Rehfeld, 1971) has made measurements of gastrin much simpler and more reliable.

To interpret the results of gastrin radioimmunoassays properly, one must understand the different forms of gastrin:

Gastrin I: Hepatadecapeptide gastrin without a sulfated tyrosine residue.

Gastrin II: Hepatadecapeptide gastrin with a sulfated tyrosine residue.

Big gastrin: Also called gastrin-34 or component II on long sephadex G-50 superfine columns (Rehfeld, 1974).

Little gastrin: Gastrin-17 or component III (Rehfeld, 1974).

Mini gastrin: Gastrin-14 or component IV.

Gastrin component I: Structure is not yet known even though the molecular size is that of proinsulin.

Big-big gastrin: Originally described by Yalow and Berson (1972) and claimed to be the major part of immunoreactive gastrin in normal fasting sera; has now been shown to be an artifact (Rehfeld et al., 1977).

Circulating gastrin is composed of components I through IV, with 90% or more being components II and III (Rehfeld, 1974).

The main tissue source of gastrin is the gastric antral mucosa (20 μg per gram of mucosa). The upper duodenum, lower duodenum, and proximal jejunum contain approximately 2 μg, 0.2 μg, and 0.1 μg per gram, respectively, of gastrin in their mucosa. In antral mucosa the main components are II and III, about 90% being component III. The C-terminal tetra peptide gastrin-4 (tetragastrin) recently was shown to be present in high concentration in the antrum (Rehfeld, 1979). Gastrin-4 is not readily measured by radioimmunoassay and is rapidly degraded in the liver. In the duodenum about 50% of mucosal gastrin is component II.

The ZE syndrome is the main clinical indication for the determination of serum gastrin levels. However, whenever serum gastrin levels are high, other causes of hypergastrinemia (Walsh, 1979) should be excluded. Moderate to extreme hypergastrinemia occurs in patients with pernicious anemia and atrophic gastritis. Patients with benign and malignant gastric ulcers, the postvagotomy state and those taking histamine H_2 receptor antagonists, anticholinergics, or antacids, may have levels of serum gastrin up to three times normal. Rarely, patients in renal failure or rheumatoid arthritis may have hypergastrinemia.

Inappropriate hypergastrinemia occurs in patients with gastrinomas, retained excluded antrum, G cell hyperplasia, pyloric stenosis with outlet obstruction, and short bowel syndrome. These conditions can usually be differentiated by clinical features and gastric acid studies in addition to gastrin determinations. It is important to know the specificity of the gastrin assay, and the antiserum used should have an equimolar potency to all gastrin components. The serum of patients with ZE syndrome does not differ, in the distribution of the various gastrin components, from that of normal or peptic ulcer patients (Rehfeld and Stadil, 1972, 1973).

Gastrin-producing tumors in the ZE syndrome are found in the pancreas, upper duodenum, and antrum; rarely in other sites (Isenberg et al., 1973; Creutzfeldt et al., 1975). Gastrinomas are usually small, multiple, slow-growing malignant tumors (Zollinger and Coleman, 1974). Often they are so small that only a large metastatic tumor in the liver, omentum of lymph node is easily diagnosed, and a small 2–3-mm primary tumor is not discovered until laparotomy (Isenberg et al., 1973; Creutzfeldt et al., 1975; Stadil and Stage, 1979). The cell of origin of pancreatic gastrinoma is disputed, since the adult pancreas does not produce gastrin, except possibly during late fetal life (Like and Orci, 1972). The D cells seem to be the most likely source of gastrin in pancreatic gastrinomas (Larsson et al., 1976). Approximately 30% of such pancreatic tumors are solitary (Ellison and Wilson, 1964); more often they are multiple. Metastases are commonly present and can be excluded only if serum gastrin levels decrease to normal after tumor extirpation. The most reliable method of diagnosing such a tumor is immunohistology, in which cells reacting with antigastrin serum are demonstrated.

Gastrinomas may produce multiple hormones (Arnold et al., 1977) such as pancreatic polypeptide, insulin, and ACTH (Larsson et al., 1975). The clinical syndrome resulting from the hyperfunction of one of the cell types in multihormonal neoplasms does not always show predominance of this cell type. Furthermore, the metastases originating from mixed tumors are not necessarily composed of the cell type responsible for the clinical picture.

Ultrastructurally, gastrinomas have been divided into four types (Creutzfeldt et al., 1975):

1. Tumors with cells containing granules typical of human antral G cells
2. Tumors with cells containing both typical and atypical G cell granules
3. Tumors containing only cells with atypical granules
4. Tumors producing multiple hormones with cells also containing the characteristic granules of other gastrointestinal endocrine cells

Most ZE tumors, though malignant, are slow growing, and long patient survival—up to 17 years—has been reported (Zollinger and Coleman, 1974). Other patients have a rapid downhill course.

Symptoms in ZE syndrome are variable and can be grouped as follows:

1. Episodic dyspeptic pain lasting for a few weeks followed by a symptom free period of up to five years (Stage and Stadil, 1979).

2. Fulminant ulcer diathesis with perforation, hemorrhage, esophagitis, and stricture within a few months after the onset.

3. Chronic ulcer disease—most commonly in the duodenal bulb or stomach. Atypical location of these ulcers such as the second, third, or fourth parts of the duodenum or jejunum and multiplicity of ulcers, even though seen in only 25% of all cases, is much more classical for ZE syndrome. In 14% of patients the ulcers are present in the distal duodenum, and 11% have jejunal ulcers. Large ulcers greater than 2 cm in diameter and two or more adjacent or widely separated ulcers should arouse suspicion of the entity. Furthermore, rapid recurrence of peptic ulcers after conventional surgery such as the occurrence of an anastomotic ulcer within two months after gastrojejunostomy or poor response to medical therapy should also lead to the suspicion of ZE syndrome. In about 20% of patients, diarrhea is the primary symptom and about 40% of patients have both diarrhea and ulcer pain.

The diagnosis of ZE syndrome is made by the demonstration of hyperchlorhydria (basal acid secretion of more than 10–15 mEq/ hour) and hypergastrinemia. About 30% of patients have associated endocrinopathies such as hyperparathyroidism, insulinoma, pituitary tumor, or adrenal cortical adenoma. First-degree relatives of the proband also have a high frequency of endocrinopathy (Lamers et al., 1978).

Radiologically, one or more ulcers, giant gastric mucosal folds, rapid intestinal transit, increased fluid content of the intestine, and a thickening of the mucosal folds in the duodenum, jejenum, and ileum are often seen. These findings can be confirmed endoscopically. A large volume of juice is usually present in the stomach.

Basal acid secretion of 20 mEq/hour or more is almost diagnostic and all patients with acid secretion above 10 mEq/hour should have a serum gastrin determination. Since gastric acid secretion in ZE is variable, multiple determinations may be necessary.

Fasting hypergastrinemia is the single most diagnostic test (Stage et al., 1978; Stage and Stadil, 1979). However, increase of serum gastrin levels to five or more times normal and acid hypersecretion

are found in only 50% of patients with the ZE syndrome. In
patients with borderline hypergastrinemia, a number of provocative
tests have been devised, including the secretin stimulation test, a
test meal (Straus et al., 1974), the calcium infusion test (Passaro
et al., 1972), the Bombesin test, and the glucagon test (Becker
et al., 1973).

In the secretin stimulation test peripheral venous blood is obtained
at 5-minute intervals for 30 to 60 minutes before and after the
intravenous administration of 1-3 units of GIH secretin per
kilogram of body weight.

In ZE syndrome, patients with a brief peak to about three times
the basal gastrin level is noted. This peak level is significantly
higher than in duodenal ulcer patients and normals. This type of
response was considered to be abnormal because secretin was
believed to lower gastrin concentrations in serum (Isenberg et al.,
1972; Kolts et al., 1974). This interpretation has been shown to be
incorrect (Stage et al., 1978). Furthermore, not all ZE patients
have such marked response. Patients with retained antrum can be
distinguished from the ZE syndrome by this test.

In the modified secretin test 1-2 U/kg is given I.V. over a 30-
second period and blood is obtained at 5, 10, 15, and 30 minutes
after injection for comparison with a sample obtained before
injection. In about 80% of patients with ZE syndrome, gastrin
rises twofold or more in 5 to 10 minutes.

The meal test is based upon the autonomous nature of hypergastrinemia in patients with ZE syndrome. Only small serum
gastrin rises are expected after a standard test meal (Straus et al.,
1974). The test is useful in diagnosing antral G-cell hyperplasia,
which is characterized by fasting hypergastrinemia and an excessive
gastrin response to feeding (Straus and Yalow, 1975). According
to Straus and Yalow (1974), a more than doubled plasma gastrin
level after a standard test meal is evidence against ZE syndrome
and consistent with the diagnosis of nontumorous hypergastrinemic
hyperchlorhydria. Such patients have insignificant responses to
secretin or calcium infusion tests.

The calcium infusion test involves measurement of serum gastrin
concentrations during infusion of 12-15 mg/kg of calcium gluconate
over three hours. In Z.E. syndrome the increase in serum gastrin is
higher than in normals and ulcer patients (Lamers and van
Tongeren, 1977), but results do overlap (Stage and Stadil, 1979).
Patients with very high basal gastrin may show poor responses to
calcium infusion. After total gastrectomy, the typical response to
this test may no longer occur even though the tumor remains. A

shorter test has been proposed in which acid secretions are measured after rapid I.V. injection of 2 mg/kg of calcium.

The Bombesin test is based on the observation that Bombesin is a potent stimulator of gastric acid secretion and plasma immunoreactive gastrin. Peak acid and gastrin responses are similar to those of a meal. Antrectomy reduces serum gastrin levels. The response in gastrin levels in antrectomized patients is absent. The Bombesin test therefore may be of value in patients with retained antrum. Since Bombesin is not generally available, the value of this test is limited at present.

In the glucagon test the patient is given 25 μg/kg of glucagon intramuscularly and blood samples are obtained every 5 minutes for 60 minutes. Some patients with ZE syndrome show a marked increase in serum gastrin levels.

The best method for differentiating ZE syndrome from duodenal ulcer disease is the measurement of basal serum gastrin concentrations, even repeatedly when one is in doubt (Stage et al., 1978). Once the diagnosis of ZE syndrome has been made, the tumor should be localized by ultrasonography, CAT scanning, peritoneoscopy, and simultaneous blood sampling for gastrin assay from pancreatic vessels and systemic veins. The new technique of percutaneous transhepatic puncture under local anesthesia (Ingemansson, 1977; Burcharth et al., 1979) with portal catheterization and venous blood sampling was recently described.

The histamine H_2 receptor antagonist cimetidine has become the treatment of choice in most cases of ZE syndrome. Dosage can be adjusted to make the patient symptom-free. Such treatment does not alter serum gastrin levels. So far the only significant side effect of long-term therapy has been gynecomastia; resistance to the drug has not developed. Thus total gastrectomy is unnecessary.

The success of medical therapy can be monitored by repeated gastric acid measurements.

Surgery still plays a role, however, in patients whose tumor growth suddenly accelerates with invasive widespread metastases (Stage et al., 1978). Almost 30% of patients in some series have such a course. Radical surgery (Whipple's operation) is possible in only a small percentage of ZE syndrome patients. In these patients the tumor has been localized before surgery and transhepatic portal vein catheterization with blood sampling for gastrin assay shows no metastatic tumor or tumors in the remaining pancreas. Five such patients, one year postoperatively, are doing well and their serum gastrin levels have remained close to zero (Burcharth et al., 1979; Stage and Stadil, 1979b). In patients with

acceleration of tumor growth streptozotocin has sometimes been
helpful (Stage and Stadil, 1979b) with temporary clinical remission
and decrease in serum gastrin levels for one to three years.

OTHER GUT ENDOCRINE TUMOR SYNDROMES

The existence of gut endocrine tumors has become well known
since the availability of radioimmunoassay for major gastrointestinal
hormones. However, since the secretory products of the majority
of endocrine cells of the gut are still unknown and not all endocrine cells have thus far been characterized in terms of their
secretory product, the list of the syndromes is incomplete. The
following symptoms and signs should alert the physician to consider
the possible presence of these tumors.
1. Diarrhea and/or steatorrhoea
2. Episodic hypoglycemia
3. Flushing
4. Bullous dermatosis
5. Diabetic glucose tolerance
6. Recurrent or ectopic peptic ulcers
7. Cushing's syndrome
8. Intestinal stasis and villous hypertrophy
9. Psychiatric disturbances otherwise unexplained
10. Hypokalemic acidosis/alkalosis

Most gut endocrine tumors, because of their histologic features,
amine precursor uptake, and decarboxylation capability, were
believed to be derived from neuroectoderm (Pearse, 1975).
Recently Pictet et al. (1976) and Le Douarin (1978) have shown
that such tumors may not originate from the neuroectoderm. A
common origin of the APUD cells from the ectoblast and a close
relationship between these cells, however, are still true.

Most tumors are classified according to their secretory product,
for example, gastrinoma or insulinoma. Mixed endocrine tumors
are difficult to classify in such a system, but no better classification
is presently available. Multiple endocrine adenopathy type I
(Wermer's syndrome) is often transmitted as an autosomal dominant, thus indicating at least a partial genetic etiology. Most gut
endocrine tumors are mixed and produce several hormones or
peptides. Especially frequent are tumors of PP cells, somatostatin
cells, and D_1 cells. In the pancreas, it is believed that most tumors
arise from the ductules that contain multipotent stem cells or

nesidioblasts that can proliferate and differentiate into various types of peptide-producing cells (Creutzfeldt, 1975; Larrson, 1978). Such multipotent stem cells or multiple types of endocrine cells, either in the same tumor or at different sites in multiple endocrine adenopathy type I, are responsible for certain unusual and unexplained clinical observations, such as:

1. Symptoms of the disease that change from one syndrome to another during treatment or over time (Broder and Carter, 1973; Hammer and Sale, 1975)

2. Metastases from gut endocrine tumor containing only some of the original cells and therefore producing a new endocrine syndrome (Larsson et al., 1975)

Since many tumors are of mixed type, it behooves the clinician to obtain levels of as many peptides as possible so that further insights into the manifestations of these syndromes can be obtained. In addition to the ZE syndrome, the following characteristic clinical syndromes are recognized.

1. The Verner-Morrison syndrome
2. The glucagonoma syndrome
3. The insulinomas
4. Somatostatinoma
5. The carcinoid syndrome
6. Multiple endocrine adenomatosis

THE VERNER-MORRISON SYNDROME

Verner and Morrison (1958) reported two patients with refractory diarrhea who died from uremia and hypokalemia and at autopsy showed solitary benign non-B islet cell adenomata of the pancreas, but no peptic ulcer. The authors postulated that the tumor cell type was different from the ZE syndrome. In 1960 Chears et al. cured a similar patient by resecting a non-B islet cell adenoma. Many names have since been given to this syndrome, including pancreatic cholera (Matsumoto et al., 1966); WDHA (watery diarrhea hypokalemia achlorhydria) syndrome (Marks et al., 1967); and WDHH (watery diarrhea, hypokalemia, hypoclorhydria) syndrome (Verner, 1968).

Clinically, the syndrome is characterized by the following features.

1. Profuse, tea-colored, episodic, cholera-like diarrhea, often of many years' duration, amounting to 6 or 8 liters per day. The

stools contain up to 20 times the normal amount of potassium per 24 hours, that is, up to 300 mEq. Eventually the diarrhea becomes sustained and relentless.

2. Hypokalemia with serum potassium levels below 3 mEq/l with a range of 1.2–3.6 mEq/l. Stool bicarbonate loss may result in acidosis during the diarrheal attacks.

3. Basal hypochlorhydria or achlorhydria in about 60% of patients, half of whom fail to respond to histamine stimulation; however, the parietal cells are normal (Kraft et al., 1969). Postoperative gastric secretory studies in some patients show a temporary rebound hyperchlorhydria and superficial peptic ulcerations suggesting that a gastric secretory inhibitory substance may have been secreted by the tumor. Hypokalemia does not seem totally to account for the hypochlorhydria as suggested by De Muro et al. (1961), since gastric achlorhydria can occur in the presence of a normal serum potassium level (Andersson et al., 1972). It seems likely that the tumor elaborates material that inhibits gastric hydrochloric acid secretion.

4. Flushing of the skin has been described by Murray et al. (1961). Such episodes are characterized by patchy erythematous and sometimes urticarial flushing. The cause is not known.

5. Glucose intolerance occurs in 50% of patients and reverts to normal after tumor extirpation. This phenomenon may result from the diabetogenic effect of tumor products or from hypokalemia.

6. Hypercalcemia is a common manifestation, cured by tumor resection, and therefore probably related to tumor secretions. Parathyroid surgery is not recommended (Brown and Crile, 1964) and, when performed, does not control the hypercalcemia.

7. Tetany has been reported in five cases (Verner and Morrison, 1958; Brown and Crile, 1964; Koenen-Schambling et al., 1970; Stoker and Wynn, 1970). Tetany usually becomes apparent when potassium replacement therapy is instituted and may be due to hypomagnesemia. However, in other diarrheal states, where serum calcium is increased or normal, tetany is rare and thus may be a diagnostic clue to the presence of the Verner-Morrison syndrome.

8. A large atonic gallbladder in older patients and gall stones in younger patients have been described (Matsumoto et al., 1966; Zenker et al., 1966; Zollinger et al., 1968). The gallbladder contains dilute bile with a fourfold or more increase in bicarbonate and chloride concentration over normal.

9. Psychosis has been reported in several patients and may have resulted from electrolyte imbalances or dehydration (Martini et al., 1964; Pabst et al., 1969).

10. Other manifestations, probably secondary to hypokalemia, include renal failure and uremia with vacuolar tubular nephropathy (the usual cause of death in untreated patients), and severe post-operative congestive failure (Lopes et al., 1970; Classen et al., 1972). The latter is rare and has been ascribed to myocardial injury secondary to hypokalemia.

The only constant feature of the Verner-Morrison syndrome is watery diarrhea, and such diarrhea can be seen in any gut endocrine tumor that is producing gastrin or calcitonin or vasoactive intestinal polypeptide or 5-hydroxytryptamine and kallikreins or prostaglandins or glucagon and gastrin or pancreatic polypeptide or substance P.

A tumor producing one or more of these peptides should be sought in patients with intractable watery diarrhea. Even apudomas that are entirely extrapancreatic, such as calcitonin-producing thyroid tumors or VIP-producing ganglioneuromas, may be responsible for such diarrhea.

Of 1000 plasma samples examined by one laboratory since 1973 (Bloom et al., 1973), 39 samples had increased VIP levels and in each case a VIP-secreting tumor was found. Seven of these tumors were outside the pancreas (ganglioneuromas or ganglioneuroblastomas). Eleven patients with the classical V.M. syndrome had normal VIP levels and no tumor. These cases were labelled as pseudo-Verner-Morrison syndrome. Other patients in this series had medullary carcinoma of the thyroid, carcinoma lung, and villous adenomas. A reliable technique to assay serum VIP levels is now available (Fahrenkrug and Schaffalitzky de Muckadell, 1977). If VIP levels in patients with intractable diarrhea are normal, screening for other peptides should be performed.

Secretin has been suggested to be the cause of diarrhea in the Verner-Morrison syndrome (Zollinger et al., 1968; Sircus et al., 1970), a claim that has not been substantiated. Even though secretin-producing cells have been located in endocrine tumors (Leupold et al., 1978; Solcia et al., 1978), increased secretin levels have not been reported in endocrine tumors. Similarly, the postulation that gastrin and glucagon together produce the intractable diarrhea in the V.M. syndrome (Barbezat and Grossman, 1971) has not been substantiated. Some authors have proposed prostaglandins to be the cause of diarrhea (Horton, 1969; Jaffe and Condon, 1976; Jaffe et al., 1977), based upon the knowledge that prostaglandin E_2 is responsible for blocking reabsorption of fluid and electrolytes in everted hamster sacs (Kaplan et al., 1970), that PGE and PGE_2 stimulate mucosal adenyl cyclase activity in rabbits in a manner similar to cholera toxin (Kimberg et al., 1971), and that prostaglandin E serves as an essential element in the system determining fluid and ion transport in the gastrointestinal tract (Rask-Madsen and Bukhave, 1979). PGE is known to inhibit intestinal motility and Rudick et al. (1970) showed that PGE_1 inhibits pancreatic secretion. On the other hand, Sircus et al. (1970) and Zollinger et al. (1968) found increased pancreatic secretion in patients with V.M. syndrome. Due to the extremely rapid synthesis of PGE, measurements of plasma PGE may actually reflect the levels of its precursor arachidonic acid rather than those of PGE and may not reflect its decreased synthesis when inhibitors of its synthesis are used in treatment (Jaffe et al., 1977). Since some patients with WDHA syndrome have flushing and skin rash, serotonin has been suggested as a cause, but without documented proof.

The main peptide thought to produce the V.M. syndrome in humans as well as pigs is VIP when plasma VIP levels exceed 90 P moles/l (Modlen et al., 1977). During streptozotocin treatment of a patient with a VIP-secreting tumor, the diarrhea stopped when VIP levels decreased below 90 P moles/l (Holst, 1979). VIP is a powerful stimulant of intestinal secretion, inhibits histamine and pentagastrin-stimulated gastric secretion, and enhances glycogenolysis. VIP levels seem to reflect the activity of the disease. However, an identical syndrome with normal VIP levels and very high serum pancreatic polypeptide levels and tumor polypeptide levels with a P Poma has been described (Fahrenkrug and Schaffalitzky de Muckadell, 1978). One should also remember that plasma VIP levels may be increased in cases of islet cell hyperplasia and advanced hepatic failure (Said, 1978).

At present VIPomas are the major cause of the watery diarrhea syndrome (WDS), but gastrinomas, prostaglandin-producing tumors, and P Pomas may also produce this syndrome. The surreptitious use of laxatives and the use of diuretics (Krejs et al., 1977) may also be associated with increased serum VIP concentrations. Tumor localization can be achieved by celiac angiography and CAT scans, selective venous samplings, and ultrasonic and nuclear imaging techniques. Occasionally, a radiographically dilated gallbladder or colon may be of diagnostic help.

The primary treatment of VIPomas consists of surgery. For unresectable or metastic carcinoma streptozotocin is administered (Kahn et al., 1975; Gagel et al., 1976; Fahrenkrug and Schaffalitzky de Muckadell, 1979). Surgery includes tumor excision and subtotal distal pancreatectomy or total pancreatectomy in cases with diffuse hyperplasia of non-B islets or microadenomatosis. Radiotherapy may be helpful for some patients.

Prognosis is usually good, and remission is achieved in 50% of patients after surgery where the tumor has not grown excessively or metastasized. In a review of 55 cases of this syndrome (Verner and Morrison, 1974), 12 patients had hyperplasia of the islets, 20 had islet tumors that were regarded as benign, and 22 had malignant tumors. One case showed no pathologic changes in the pancreas.

THE GLUCAGONOMA SYNDROME

The first documented case of a glucagon secreting malignant islet cell carcinoma was a 42-year-old female with bullous and eczematoid dermatitis and mild maturity-onset diabetes, described by McGavran et al. (1966). This patient had an A-cell carcinoma histologically and high tumor and blood levels of glucagon. Injection of glucagon obtained from the tumor increased the blood glucose level by 46 mg% in a dog. Glucagon-producing tumors were described in some detail in 1974 (Croughs, 1974) but recognition of the glucagonoma syndrome must be credited to Mallinson et al. (1974). The syndrome is characterized by the following features.

1. Necrolytic migratory erythema: This consists of bullous lesions with intra- and intercellular edema in the epidermis corresponding to the stratum granulosum and lucidum with necrosis and has been recognized as an entity since 1942 (Becker et al., 1942). More recent descriptions are those of Wilkinson (1973) and Sweet (1974). It appears that all cases of this skin rash so far reported have been associated with pancreatic tumors and a clinical picture compatible with glucagonoma syndrome. The bullous dermatosis is clinically seen as erosions and crusts in the area of perineum, groin, gluteal regions, distal part of the extremities, and central face. Some patients have scaly plaques and papules. The skin rash is intermittent and is subject to change when superinfection occurs. The pathogenesis of rash is not clear and it appears that persistently elevated glucagon levels may not be causative. In patients receiving large doses of glucagon for a long time similar rash has not developed. Other metabolic products from the tumor may be causative. A recent one-case study suggests that the skin rash is most likely due to an amino acid deficiency and can be rapidly reversed by total parenteral nutrition (Norton et al., 1979). The rash, however, seems to be the most important diagnostic clue, even though often a late one, when the tumor has already spread.

2. Hypoaminoacidemia: Plasma amino acid concentrations in this syndrome are considerably lower than normal; this occurs

more often than a diabetic glucose tolerance. It has been shown previously that high glucagon levels in blood have only transient effects on blood glucose but a more persistent effect on blood amino acids (Marliss et al., 1970).

3. Diabetic glucose tolerance or diabetes mellitus: Because experimentally induced hyperglucagonemia has only transitory effects on blood glucose and glucose tolerance (Sherwin et al., 1976; Holst et al., 1977; Holst, 1978), it should be emphasized that lack of glucose intolerance does not exclude this condition, even though the glucose intolerance is a more common finding.

4. Thromboembolic complications are rather frequent in this condition and may be pulmonary or elsewhere. The onset of these complications in a patient with skin lesions of bullous nature resistant to therapy should lead to an urgency in diagnosis in this otherwise slowly progressive neoplastic syndrome, since these embolic phenomena pose a serious threat to the life of the patient.

5. Other nonspecific features:
   (a) Weight loss
   (b) Anemia usually normocytic normochromic
   (c) Atrophic glossitis
   (d) Cheilitis angularis
   (e) Psychiatric disturbances
   (f) Hypersedimentation
   (g) Neurologic manifestations

In a patient clinically suspected to have this syndrome, on the basis of the features outlined, plasma glucagon levels should be determined and are usually five to ten times the normal values, the typical levels being 300–1000 pg/ml. The glucagon secretion may or may not be suppressed by glucose infusions; similarly, arginine infusions (A-cell secretagogue) do not always stimulate glucagon production in these cases (Holst, 1978). Somatostatin has been shown to inhibit glucagon secretion in two cases (Mortimer et al., 1974; Holst and Ingemansson, 1976) and the pancreatic and hepatic responses to exogenous glucagon are blunted. It should be realized, however, that since glucagon and amino acid determinations are not routinely available these cases are most likely to be found by the dermatologists, who in cases of therapy-resistant bullous dermatosis should obtain plasma glucagon analysis.

Once the diagnosis has been made preoperative localization of the tumor can proceed by selective catheterization of pancreatic veins and analyzing the samples for hormones. Hepatic deposits may be located by hepatic vein catheterization (Ingemansson, 1977). Selective angiography, ultrasonography, and CAT scanning may also be helpful.

Glucagonoma as part of the polyglandular adenomata syndrome has been described (Croughs et al., 1972): the patient had an adreno-cortical adenoma with Cushing's syndrome, an enlarged parathyroid gland with hypercalcemia and a glucagonoma. Another case reported recently developed diabetic ketoacidosis (Domen et al., 1980).

Histologic interpretation of glucagonomas so far has been of a primitive nature, because usual islet cell staining techniques for normal islets are not suitable for tumor cells and cell recognition by secretory products (immunocytochemistry) is necessary to identify other constituents of these tumors and their role in the clinical picture.

The treatment of the tumor in early stages is surgical removal that may be curative. Where enucleation of the tumor is not feasible, the tail of the pancreas may be resected (Ingemansson, 1977). Streptozotocin treatment has been tried in this condition (Danforth et al., 1976) but the results are not promising. Death usually occurs in untreated cases by extreme debilitation or thromboembolic complications. Rash may be treated symptomatically (Pedersen et al., 1976).

THE INSULINOMAS

Insulinomas are tumors that secrete insulin and proinsulin and cause hypoglycemia. The majority of them are found in the pancreas but approximately 2% may originate in ectopic pancreatic tissue, usually adjacent to the pancreas. Wilder et al. (1927) first described this tumor. A variety of other neoplasms may produce hypoglycemia by different mechanisms, some of them not too well understood, but do not produce insulin or proinsulin and therefore are not insulinomas.

Insulinomas are rare tumors and very few statistics on their incidence or prevalence are available. In Seattle 21 cases of insulinoma were seen by Kavlie and White (1972), giving an annual incidence of one case per 1×10^6 people. From Radcliffe infirmary, Oxford, one case per 5×10^5 persons per year was reported (Keynes, 1970).

Insulinoma is slightly more common in females than in males, and the average age at diagnosis is in the early to mid-forties, even though the tumor has been diagnosed in a newborn (Salinas et al., 1968) and in an 80-year-old (Miller, 1965). However, such an occurrence is clearly unusual.

Clinically, patients with insulinoma present v.ith episodes of spontaneous hypoglycemia of a subacute and chronic nature (Marks and Rose, 1965). Altered behavior and disturbances of consciousness are common and almost any neurologic or psychiatric condition may be simulated. The symptoms usually are of many months or years in duration. In their ten patients the average duration of symptoms was 3.8 years in the series of Tompkins et al. (1967). Intellectual and motor impairment is often mistaken for severe alcohol intoxication during subacute episodes. The symptoms of hypoglycemia are characteristically seen before breakfast or lunch or after excessive exertion and are present for many years. Patients are usually obese because of the necessity to alleviate the symptoms of hypoglycemia. The florid manifestations of acute hypoglycemia are seldom seen. In chronic cases personality changes, poor memory, psychosis, and dementia are all seen. Rarely, polyneuropathy and progressive muscular atrophy may be encountered.

Insulinomas may develop as part of Wermer's (MEA I) pluriglandular syndrome, and there is some indication that familial occurrence of diabetes mellitus may be associated with that of insulinoma. In a strain of hereditary diabetic mice (Like et al., 1965), insulinomas develop frequently, tending to ameliorate diabetes. A high familial incidence is reported in a series of 80 cases of insulinomas in which about 30% had a family history of diabetes (Priestly, 1962). Of 55 diabetic patients treated with sulfonylureas and studied at postmortem, four had islet cell tumors (Balodimos et al., 1968).

Most insulinomas are solitary benign tumors 5-50 cm in diameter found throughout the pancreas. Diffuse adenomatosis of islets is seen in about 4% of cases and existence of generalized hyperplasia of all the islets has been postulated in some cases. Less than 5% of the insulinomas metastasize, generally to the liver (Stefanini et al., 1974).

Histologically, insulinomas are impossible to distinguish from other peptide-secreting tumors of the pancreas. However, by immunohistology using insulin antiserum 90% of tumors react, while those with insulin concentrations below 1.0/g tissue give a negative immunohistologic reaction. Ultrastructurally, the tumors have been classified into four types (Creutzfeldt et al., 1973).

Type I: Those containing typical beta granules
Type II: Those containing both typical and atypical granules
Type III: Those containing only atypical granules
Type IV: Those with virtually agranular cells

Insulinoma cells contain less insulin than normal human B-cells, and no tumor has been shown to contain more insulin than the normal pancreas. Hyperinsulinism in insulinoma patients therefore does not appear to be due to insulin overproduction. However, the proinsulin concentrations seemed to be increased, the highest being in Type IV tumors. The decreased storage capacity thus may be responsible for an uncontrolled insulin release in some tumor cells.

It may be important to remind the reader that insulin is synthesized in the endoplasmic reticulum of the B-cells as a precursor proinsulin (Taylor, 1972). The proinsulin is then transformed into insulin and the connecting C chain by proteolytic cleavage in the golgi complex. They are then incorporated into the B granules. Proinsulin has a molecular weight of approximately 9000 and constitutes about 2.5% of the total immunoreactive insulin (IRI) in normal pancreatic islets, as against up to 14% in the insulinoma tissue. Proinsulin generally constitutes less than 25% of the total plasma IRI. It is only 10–25% as active as insulin and is not converted to insulin outside the pancreas. Proinsulin levels are highest during fasting, because conventional stimulation releases only insulin, and not proinsulin, from the pancreas.

Diagnosis of insulinoma depends upon demonstration of hypoglycemia (blood glucose in the 40–50-mg range) during fasting (overnight fast of 15 hours, but with free access to water). This should be repeated at least three times. Prolonged fasts of 72 hours or more, though suggested, are not always diagnostic (Power, 1969). Normal subjects and those with fasting hypoglycemia attributable to other causes show depression of peripheral plasma insulin levels to less than 10 μu/ml during fasting-provoked hypoglycemia. Under these circumstances patients with insulinomas show normal or raised plasma insulin levels, a clearly inappropriate insulin response. These observations lead to a simple, nonaggressive, and most reliable diagnostic test for insulinoma: the four-hourly repeated evaluation of the ratio of the plasma concentration of immunoreactive insulin (in microunits per milliliter) to the concentration of plasma glucose (in milligrams per deciliter)—IRI/G ratio—during a 16- to 24-hour fast. An IRI/G ratio curve ascending beyond 0.30 is diagnostic for insulinoma, while normal individuals and patients with hypoglycemia of other etiologies will show an IRI/G ratio curve descending much below 0.30 (Fajans and Floyd, 1976; Merimee, 1977). Furthermore, a fasting blood sample, when analyzed for proinsulin, insulin, C-peptide, and glucose, always reveals high levels of proinsulin in insulinoma (Turner and Heding, 1977; Faber and Kehlet, 1979), if uremia, liver cirrhosis, and thyrotoxicosis are excluded. In surreptitious insulin administration one may also see hyperproinsulinemia, but insulin levels are high when compared with simultaneous C-peptide levels. Hypoglycemia attributable to sulfonylureas is characterized by a proportionate elevation of all three. When all three of these—namely, proinsulin, insulin, and C-peptide—are low in a hypoglycemic patient, other causes must be sought.

Other tests to demonstrate inappropriate insulin secretion when a patient is not hypoglycemic have been devised. Such tests include the alcohol infusion test (Turner et al., 1973), which depresses hepatic glucose release without stimulating endogenous insulin secretion, or use of fish insulin (Turner and Johnson, 1973), which has the biological but not the immunologic properties of the human insulin. These tests still may miss occasional insulinomas that secrete insulin only episodically.

A glucose-calcium infusion test (Frerichs and Creutzfeldt, 1976) using 5 mg/kg/hr Ca^{++} for three hours, during and after a one-hour glucose infusion, potentiates glucose-induced insulin release, in insulinoma, hence increases serum insulin levels and causes a much faster blood glucose fall at the end of the glucose infusion. Such an exaggerated insulin response is not seen in normals and after surgery for insulinomas.

Suppression of inappropriate insulin secretion in response to i.v. infusion of 600 mg diazoxide over a one-hour period in a hypo-glycemic subject helps confirm that IRI is due to pancreatic insulin and gives some indication of the therapeutic effectiveness of diazoxide, in case a tumor is not located at surgery. Some tumors, especially those in children, may not be diazoxide responsive.

Many other tests previously used in the diagnosis of insulinomas aimed at stimulating insulin release without provoking fasting hypo-glycemia, such as tolbutamide, glucagon, glucose, leucine, and arginine tests, have not proved consistently reliable, and with the advent of simultaneous radioimmunoassay for insulin, proinsulin, and C-peptide, have become mostly useless. Caerulein, from toad skin, also stimulates insulin release from insulinoma patients, but has no effect in normals (Fallucca et al., 1972). Where the presence of insulinoma is chemically suspected the tumor may be localized by celiac axis and superior mesenteric angiography. Some series claim a success rate of 75% (Alfidi et al., 1971) or higher (Boijsen and Samuelsson, 1970). However, on an average, the success rate is probably around 30%. The variable vascularity and the small size may be responsible factors. It should be remembered, however, that islet hyperplasia in nesidioblastoma may be responsible for cases of pernicious hyperinsulinemia and in infants may cause neonatal hypoglycemia or sudden death (Larsson, 1978; Polak et al., 1978; Welbourn et al., 1978). Both diazoxide and extensive pancreatic resection may be needed for treatment. New potent long-acting somatostatin analogues may be useful in this entity, thus avoiding brain injury before definitive treatment can be established.

From a therapeutic point of view, insulinomas are cured by surgery, whereas medical treatment is only symptomatic. Recently, Stefanini et al. (1974) received 1067 cases of B islet cell tumors, 925 of which were obtained from an international inquiry. On the basis of this study, they concluded that early surgery should be the treatment of choice. In the tumors of the body and tail, distal resection rather than local excision is preferable because of fewer complications and the occassional advantage of removing an additional occult lesion. In occult tumors progressive resection from left to right is advised, the extent of resection being guided by pathologic examination of each portion of pancreas removed, and simultaneous intraoperative blood sugar levels. As far as possible, every effort should be made to localize the tumor pre-operatively, and intraoperatively if need be, but the tumor should be removed at the first operation to avoid subsequent fistulas and pseudocysts. Blind progressive pancreatic resection can be applied also to cases of islet hyperplasia. Operative mortality was 11% in this large series. If the techniques of CT scanning and selective venous samplings are available, the tumor may be precisely localized preoperatively and should make blind progressive resections of the pancreas unnecessary.

SOMATOSTATINOMA

These tumors, only very recently described and recognized, are characterized by: (1) diabetic glucose tolerance test; (2) maldigestion, diarrhea, and steatorrhoea; (3) hypochlorhydria; and (4) tumor cells resembling normal D-cells of the pancreas. The first case was described by Larsson et al. (1977) and the second by Ganda et al. (1977) shortly thereafter. In both of these cases the tumor was discovered during a cholecystectomy, and extremely high tumor tissue and hepatic and pancreatic vein blood levels of RIA somatostatin were noted. The tumor in Ganda et al.'s case had 301 ng/mg of tissue levels of somatostatin as compared with 0.6 ng/mg tissue somatostatin levels in seven insulinomas and two glucagonomas. After resection the patient became euglycemic. Both of these patients were females, 46 and 55 years old respectively. The tumor in one case was cultured in monolayers, which remained viable for 51 days and released somatostatin into the culture medium. Since 1977 other cases have been described (De

Nutte et al., 1978; Larsson, 1978) and one case had manifested an
ectopic ACTH syndrome (Kovacs et al., 1977). In many cases
tumors have had associated PP cell hyperplasia, and this may have
been responsible for some clinical manifestations. In one case
intravenous tolbutamide greatly increased concentration of
somatostatin in plasma and may hold a diagnostic promise in future
(De Nutte et al., 1978). The tumors are slow growing and
metastasize to the liver or adjacent structures. High somatostatin
levels have been found in peripheral plasma more recently, and
even a case of somatostatinoma arising from the duodenum has
been described (Kaneko et al., 1979).

THE CARCINOID SYNDROME

The term *Karzenoide* (carcinoid) was first used in 1907 by
Oberndorfer for a group of tumors of the intestine that were slow
growing and benign. Later it was recognized that many of these
tumors had silver staining properties and so were called argentaf-
finomas. These tumors produce a fairly typical clinical syndrome
now widely recognized as the carcinoid syndrome. Extensive
reviews of all aspects of the carcinoid syndrome have been published (Grahame Smith, 1972, 1974) and this brief discussion is
intended to remind the reader of the salient points about the
syndrome.

Carcinoid tumors can be found anywhere in the gastrointestinal
tract except the esophagus. The appendix is the most common
site but the appendiceal tumors rarely produce the syndrome unless
they have metastasized. Ileal tumors are common and produce
carcinoid syndrome; gastric and jejunal tumors do so rarely. Rectal
tumors rarely produce the syndrome. Carcinoid tumors in the
ileum are often multiple and 1.5–3.5 cm in size, and usually are
asymptomatic. Only when the tumor gets too large, does one see
intestinal obstruction, intussuception, and surface ulceration with
gastrointestinal bleeding. The production of this syndrome in
association with gastrointestinal carcinoids depends upon the
presence of metastases in the liver. Only rarely does one see the
syndrome in a large mass of retroperitoneal tumor or pulmonary
metastases. The reason is that liver effectively metabolizes and
inactivates the primary tumor secretions, but when liver has
metastases they drain these products into the systemic circulation
via hepatic veins and the inactivation in the liver is avoided. The
large size of hepatic metastases may also be contributory.

Carcinoid tumors have been described in gallbladder and Meckel's diverticulum, and sometimes the primary site is hard to find. Malignant neoplasms elsewhere are found with greater frequency in patients harboring carcinoids (Moertel et al., 1961).

Carcinoids metastasize to mesenteric and posterior abdominal wall lymph nodes, ovaries, and bones, in addition to the liver; while most metastases to the bones are osteoblastic, gastric carcinoids produce osteosclerotic metastases.

Clinical Presentation

The carcinoid is an uncommon tumor. The age varies from 18 years to 76 years, and both sexes are equally affected. The tumor is slow growing and may be many years in hiding before the clinical syndrome is detected. The bronchial, pancreatic, and gastric carcinoids producing the syndrome tend to be nonmalignant. The following are the common symptoms and signs.

Flushing: Four types of flushing have been described in this syndrome (Grahame Smith, 1972), depending upon the area of the body affected (normal flushing area—face, neck, and upper anterior chest, or more widespread), the duration of the flush (2 minutes to hours), the color of the flush (erythematous, violaceous, etc.), and other associated features such as telengiectasia, Campbell du Morgan spots, hypotension, and diarrhea. The flushes associated with bronchial carcinoids are particularly prolonged and there may be associated hypotension or worsening of the diarrhea during the flush. Gastric carcinoids produce a bright red and patchy histamine flush. Cheese, bacon, alcohol, excitement, norephinephrine, or epinephrine may precipitate a flush. Alcohol and catecholamine-induced flush can be blocked by alpha-adrenergic blocking agents. Flushing is mediated by bradykinin release (Adamson et al., 1969).

Diarrhea: The severity of diarrhea (one to 20 bowel movements per day), as well as its temporal relationship to flushing, is variable. A striking dissociation often exists and leads one to think about their chemical mediation being independent. Current evidence, still inconclusive, seems to incriminate 5HT as causative for diarrhea. Methysergide, a 5HT antagonist, and parachlorophenylalanine, which inhibits the synthesis of 5HT, are both effective in controlling the diarrhea. Some pain in the abdomen is often associated with severe diarrhea.

Malabsorption: Though uncommon, malabsorption has been reported in carcinoid syndrome. The pathogenetic mechanisms involved are probably mesenteric arterial ischemia or lymphatic obstruction by tumor or fibrosis. Rarely, ileal resection may be responsible. However, jejunal mucosal biopsy is normal.

Abdominal Pain: This can be due to one of the following.

1. Peptic ulcer—an association with carcinoid syndrome is not clear cut.
2. Biliary obstruction—occurs rarely.
3. Intestinal obstruction—due to tumor or tumor-associated fibrosis.

The primary carcinoid tumors usually are not large enough to produce obstruction and usually either the fibrosis in the area of the tumor before or after surgery or muscle hypertrophy is the responsible mechanism.

4. Hepatic metastases—especially those near the surface of the liver, may undergo necrosis with elevated 5-hydroxyindole levels, tenderness in the liver, atypical abdominal pain, and friction rub on the liver.
5. Intestinal infarction—sometimes occurs in carcinoid syndrome and may cause pain.

Pulmonary Symptoms:

1. Hyperventilation—usually is seen during episodes of flushing; 5HT release may be associated.
2. Asthma—usually seems to occur, in patients who have prior chronic obstructive lung disease, during an episode of flush. It should never be treated with epinephrine. Intravenous methysergide is effective.

Fibrosis: Peritoneal fibrosis, pleural adhesions, constrictive pericarditis, and retroperitoneal fibrosis leading to urethral obstruction are all known to occur in carcinoid syndrome.

Cardiac Disease: In carcinoid syndrome cardiac involvement consists of focal or diffuse fibrosis on the luminal surface of the internal elastic lamina and young collagen can be identified on electron microscopy in these areas, more often, in the right heart. Pulmonary stenosis is usually the predominant lesion; the tricuspid valve is often fixed and usually shows regurgitation. The distribution of lesions, usually in the right heart, can be explained by the fact that some substance is released by the hepatic metastases into the hepatic veins, travels to the right heart via inferior vena cava, and in the right heart causes the damage and is probably removed in its passage through the lungs. In patients with bronchial carcinoids, metastases may drain directly into the pulmonary veins and the left heart and only left-sided heart lesions may be present.

Pellagra-like skin lesions: Are also frequently seen in this syndrome.

From a diagnostic point of view, the demonstration of increased
5 HIAA excretion in urine, exceeding 30 mg per day, provided
care is taken to avoid certain drugs (glycerylguaicolate, chlorpromazine, etc.) and certain foods (such as pineapple, walnuts,
bananas) that interfere with the chemical estimation, is a simple
screening test. The 5 HTP and 5 HT levels in urine and blood,
respectively, may occasionally be helpful, particularly when 5
HIAA excretion is normal or very slightly elevated. Quantitative
urinary 5-hydroxytryptamine higher than 1-2 mg/24 hours, in a
patient with carcinoid syndrome, indicates that tumor is a variant,
probably derived from stomach (embryonic fore gut), which
releases the serotonin precursor 5-hydroxytryptophan.

Once the diagnosis has been biochemically established, the site
of primary and metastatic tumor may be determined by barium
X-rays of the gastrointestinal tract, isotope scans of the liver,
CAT scanning, chest X-ray, bronchoscopy, pelvic examination (the
latter two to rule out a bronchial or ovarian carcinoid), and even a
liver biopsy. Carcinoid flush may be provoked by giving 5-10 μg of
epinephrine i.v. This should be avoided in patients with cardiac
failure, arrhythmias, or asthma.

Carcinoid tumors are slow growing and the patients may live
for 5-20 years with ileal and other gastrointestinal primaries and
liver metastases. In contrast, patients with bronchial and pancreatic
carcinoids live from a few months to two years. Cardiac failure,
electrolyte problems from severe diarrhea, and cachexia are usual
causes of death.

The treatment of bronchial, ovarian, or other primaries may be
surgical removal resulting in cure. Usually, however, hepatic
metastases are present by the time the clinical syndrome is
recognized. In some of these cases partial hepatectomy may
relieve or eliminate most of the symptoms. Because the dangers of
anesthesia and surgery are increased and a "carcinoid crisis" may
occur, these patients should be preoperatively treated with serotonin
antagonists such as methysergide maleate or cyproheptadine.
Prolonged postoperative hypotension may require metaraminol
bitartarate or angiotensin.

The symptomatic therapy includes the following. (1) Inhibitors
of serotonin synthesis, for example, parachlorophenylalanine 3-4
g/day maximum in divided doses, may help nausea, vomiting, and
diarrhea, and reduce the intensity of flushes. (2) Serotonin
antagonists, for example, methysergide maleate 6-24 mg daily
orally, is more effective against diarrhea than cyproheptadine.
Cyproheptadine, 6-30 mg/day orally, seems to control the flush
better. (3) Antihistamines control the flush in rare patients who

have elevated blood histamine levels. (4) Phenoxybenzamine, 10-30 mg/daily, may diminish flushing by preventing kallikrein release. Cytotoxic drug therapy using 5-fluorouracil, cyclophosphamide, and more recently streptozotocin, has been unrewarding. Radiotherapy, 4000-4500 rads, may relieve pain from bony metastases. Other therapy is basically supportive and symptomatic. Carcinoid tumors may be associated with pancreatic tumors or insulin-producing tumors and occasionally hyperpigmentation seen in carcinoid patients may be due to an excess of melanocyte-stimulating hormone production. These should be looked for and treated. More recently, intraarterial (hepatic artery) irradiation by [90] yttrium (Simon et al., 1968) using 15-20 μci of [90] yttrium and yttrium implantation in hypophysis have also been tried (Geffroy, 1967; Page, 1967), based on the theory that experimentally the light cell system is receptive to somatotrophic hormone and hypophysis destruction is useful in reducing the size of neoplastic metastases of breast and prostate, but without much success.

MULTIPLE ENDOCRINE ADENOMATOSIS (MEA)

Included under this term are a group of usually familial syndromes in which hyperplasia or tumor formation occurs in two or more endocrine glands. Two patterns are recognized:

Type I (Wermer's syndrome), in which pancreas, parathyroid, and pituitary glands are usually involved.

Type II (Sipple's syndrome), in which hyperparathyroidism, medullary carcinoma of thyroid, and pheochromocytoma are usually seen. Type II is furt`er subdivisible (Block et al., 1975). Type IIa consists of medullary thyroid carcinoma, pheochromocytoma, and parathyroid adenoma or hyperplasia. Type IIb (also called Type III) includes medullary thyroid carcinoma, pheochromocytoma, marfanoid body habitus, and mucosal neuromas, but no parathyroid disease.

In Type I, pancreatic islet cells are involved in more than 80% of cases, and gastrinomas, insulinomas, and VIPomas are found, in that order of frequency (Welbourne et al., 1978). Only occasionally are they of other types. Looking at it the other way around, at least 20 to 30% of those with gastrinomas have other endocrine tumors (Bonfils and Bernades, 1974) compared with only 4% of those with insulinomas (Stefanini et al., 1974).

The occurrence of multiple endocrine adenopathy reemphasizes the apud concept and often the "apudomas," that is, the hyperplastic or neoplastic lesions of apud cells, more clearly display the apud features than their parent cells. Apudomas arising from the endocrine (apud) cells in the islets and those between the acinar cells have been classified (Welbourne et al., 1978) as follows:

1. Orthoendocrine: Secrete the normal peptide product
   - (a) Insulinoma   (B-cell)
   - (b) Glucagonoma   (A-cell)
   - (c) Somatostatinoma   (D-cell)
   - (d) VIPoma   (D_1-cell)
   - (e) PPoma   (D_2-PP-cell)

2. Paraendocrine: Secrete amines, peptides, or other substances normally produced by other glands or tissues, but not pancreas. The cell types for these are not usually attributable or similar to other endocrine cells and the classification, therefore, is based on function (secretion). These are
   - (a) Zollinger-Ellison syndrome   (gastrin)
   - (b) Cushing's syndrome   (ACTH/CRH)
   - (c) Pigmentation   (MSH)
   - (d) Schwartz-Bartter syndrome   (ADH)
   - (e) Hypercalcemia   (PTH)
   - (f) Diarrhea   (5HT)
   - (g) Hypertension   (catecholamines)

3. Multiple hormone-secreting lesions: Frequently pancreatic apudomas secrete more than one humoral agent. Nearly all combinations of orthoendocrine and paraendocrine secretions with as many as six have been reported in one tumor. For reasons so far unknown, the clinical syndromes usually are caused by one humoral agent, the others remaining silent, which is in marked contrast to MEA patients.

GASTROINTESTINAL HORMONES

Role in GI Tract Diseases

Gastrointestinal hormones play a role in motor, secretory, and absorptive functions of the gut, even though the physiologic role of many of these peptides has not yet been defined. However, some of these functions will be briefly discussed in the context of their clinical importance:

Gastroesophageal reflux: Effects of gastrin, cholecystokinin, caerulein, secretin, glucagon, VIP, GIP, motilin, substance P, bombesin, somatostatin, and pancreatic polypeptide on lower esophageal sphincter in different species have been studied. The sum of evidence at present suggests that although gastrin may have an influence in determining lower esophageal sphincter pressure, this influence is not a major factor and other neural and hormonal influences are more important. Of the clinical studies in patients with esophageal reflux, only one of three seems to correlate hypogastrinemia with lower esophageal sphincter hypotension (Farrell et al., 1974; Lipshultz et al., 1974; Sturdevant and Kun, 1974). Lower esophageal sphincter (LES) pressure rose less in response to increasing doses of i.v. pentagastrin producing physiologic serum levels in patients with esophageal reflux than in normal subjects. Integrated gastrin output in reflux patients in response to a protein meal was also less, suggesting a deficient gastrin release. Lower pressures in LES are found in patients with pernicious anemia even though there is hypergastrinemia, and in ZE patients fasting serum gastrin levels correlate only loosely with LES pressure.

CCK, caerulein, secretin, glucagon, glucagon-like immuno-reactively (GLI), and VIP all cause a fall of LES pressure but do not have a significant role in health or disease.

Motilin, substance P, and Bombesin contract the gut smooth muscles in humans. Motilin causes phasic changes in esophageal sphincter pressure at infusion rates that may be physiologic and therefore may have a role in esophageal reflux.

Prostaglandin E_1, E_2, and A_2 in opposum and E_2 given to healthy subjects and patients with achalasia relax LES, while prostaglandin F_2 increases LES pressure. The role of prostaglandins as well as histamine and serotonin remains to be defined.

Dumping Syndrome: A considerably enhanced release of neurotensin has been shown in postoperative dumping syndrome after ulcer surgery (Blackburn et al., 1978) and may explain the fall in blood pressure and rise in hematocrit as well as late hypoglycemia seen in these patients. Also in patients with jejunoileal bypass, neurotensin levels are increased and may be due to rapid arrival of food in the terminal ileum where most of it is released by NT cells (Bloom et al., 1978).

Duodenal Ulcer Disease: The role of gastrin in ZE syndrome and retained antrum is clearly established. It is in simple duodenal ulcer disease that the role is not so clear. The role of various hormones in duodenal ulcer disease as presently understood can be summarized as follows:

Gastrin: 1. There exists a group of duodenal ulcer patients who have hypergastrinemia and excessive gastric acid production but no gastrinoma; they have increased G-cell density in the antrum and have been labeled as cases of antral G-cell hyperplasia. Theoretically, antrectomy would be curative. However, many of these patients had undergone a vagotomy earlier and this procedure raises the antral G-cell count (Malmstrom et al., 1977). This entity, if it exists, must be very rare.

2. Fasting plasma gastrins are similar in normal and duodenal ulcer patients, but in response to protein meal peak plasma gastrins are higher in patients.

3. Basal acid output and fasting plasma gastrins are not necessarily inversely proportional (Cowley et al., 1973), even though maximal acid output after meals or pentagastrin shows this relationship both in normals and patients.

4. In duodenal ulcer disease G-cell response to a mucosal stimulus (such as acid inhibition after a meal) may be intact but the neural control of G-cell may be defective (insulin-stimulated release of acid correlates with G-cell density).

Cholecystokinin: In D.U. patients there is a rapid rise in serum CCK after food (Rayford et al., 1975), this could be due to rapid emptying since similar phenomena has been noted in dumping syndrome.

Bombesin: Antral acidification fails to inhibit gastrin and gastric acid output in D.U. patients but not in normals; this effect could be due to excess Bombesin either locally or in blood, since gastrin release due to Bombesin is also not inhibited by antral acidification. More Bombesin cells have been found in duodenal biopsies in D.U. patients (McCrossan et al., 1977) than controls.

Secretin: Even if it is released by a meal, the amounts are insufficient to inhibit gastric acid and hence has no role. The effect of IV secretin in inhibiting meal-stimulated acid is the same in D.U. and normals.

Somatostatin: 1. The D-cells producing this hormone lie in the lower third of the antral mucosa below the G-cells. In one case (Polak et al., 1977) with duodenal ulcer these cells were deficient.

2. Lower D-cell concentrations by mucosal radioimmunoassay were shown in 28 D.U. patients when compared with 15 controls (Chayvialle et al., 1978).

3. In pharmacologic doses gastric acid, pepsin, and plasma gastrin responses both in fasting and stimulated state are suppressed by somatostatin, but the inhibition is less in D.U. patients, suggesting that there may be a deficiency of this local inhibitory peptide.

Motilin: Levels are not different in D.U. patients from controls.

GIP—Glucagon: Levels are not different from normals.

Whether enterogastrone or bulbogastrone released from duodenum or small intestine are important remains to be elucidated. The role of VIP in patients with duodenal ulcer has not been

looked into. Recently, it has been shown that there is an increased
PP release in humans in duodenal ulcer disease and truncal
vagotomy as well as gastrectomy result in a marked diminution of
PP response to food (Hansky et al., 1978).

Celiac Disease: In this disease, characterized by severe malabsorption and intestinal villous atrophy, the following hormonal
disturbances have been noted.

1. Poor gallbladder contractibility leading to reduced or
absent basal bile output; stagnation of bile in the biliary tree,
and hence a reduced enterohepatic circulation; reduced gut
motility; and impaired ileal absorption of bile salts resulting in a
twofold to threefold increase in taurocholate pool and prolongation
of its half-life.

2. Reduced exocrine pancreatic response to a standard meal
with diminished lipase and amylase output even though no evidence
of pancreatic insufficiency is discernible (Novis et al., 1972).

The studies so far done in celiac patients have only shown an
impaired response in serum levels of CCK and secretin after fatty
meal and acid stimulation, respectively, even though the fasting
CCK levels are high (Lowbeer et al., 1975) and those for secretin
are normal (O'Connor et al., 1977). It is not clear whether the
target organ response is poor or if stimulus for hormone output
is inadequate. In celiac children immunohistochemical studies
have shown an increase of up to 60% in the number of secretin
immunoreactive cells in duodenal crypts (Polak et al., 1973). This
observation, coupled with the fact that exogenous secretin infusion
produces normal bicarbonate secretion and luminal pH change,
would suggest a defect of storage or release of secretin in celiac
disease. The target organ responsiveness to CCK is more difficult
to assess, because defective response of pancreas and gallbladder
could also result from protein malnutrition or disuse atrophy
secondary to a lack of CCK and secretin, since both of these may
be trophic hormones.

Suffice it to say that the hormonal abnormalities described could
impair micelle formation and fat absorption. However, they are not
likely to be responsible for protein and carbohydrate
malabsorption.

Chronic Pancreatitis: hPP release in response to a meal as well as
to insulin-induced hypoglycemia is impaired in patients with
chronic pancreatitis (18-25% of normal) and may provide an
estimate of exocrine as well as endocrine function (Sive et al.,
1978; Valenzuela et al., 1978).

Diarrheal States: In infective diarrhea, tropical sprue and
Crohn's disease associated with diarrhea motilin levels are con-

siderably high and improve with successful treatment (Bloom
et al., 1978).

Intestinal Adaptation after small bowel resection: After extensive
resections of small intestine for Crohn's disease, mesenteric ischemia,
trauma, or other surgical conditions, gastric hypersecretion and
small bowel mucosal hyperplasia distal to the site of resection are
noted, and, at least in experimental animals, there is a numerical
increase in the cells in crypts as well as villi. Recently, the role of
gastrointestinal hormones in this condition has been explored and
will be reviewed.

Gastrin: This is a trophic hormone for the entire GI tract,
liver, and pancreas, with the exception of the esophagus and gastric
antrum. It is further confirmed by the gastric mucosal atrophy seen
after antrectomy and the mucosal hyperplasia seen in the ZE syndrome. Furthermore, jejunal resection causing gastric hypersecretion and parietal cell hyperplasia is associated with increased serum
gastrin. Parenterally administered, pentagastrin produces similar
results and increased DNA synthesis can be shown in the fundus
when gastrin is infused in dogs (Willems et al., 1972). However,
there are some loose ends. Hypergastrinemia seen after vagotomy
and pyloroplasty is followed by gastric mucosal atrophy and is
hard to explain (Helander, 1976). The response to gastrin, so well
seen in the stomach and duodenum, does not appear to be significant in intestinal adaptation. However, the role of luminal gastrin
has not been evaluated in physiologic amounts in humans.

Enteroglucagon: Increased plasma enteroglucagon-like
immunoreactivity in a patient with renal tumor has been described,
in which intestinal mucosal hyperplasia was present and may have a
role in intestinal adaptation after resection (Gleeson et al., 1971).
Similar findings are noted in glucagon-producing pancreatic tumors,
although an opposite effect occurs in rats small intestine (Rudo
et al., 1976) with glucagon infusion.

CCK: This is weakly trophic for stomach, and increases
pancreatic RNA, DNA, and protein synthesis, but seems to play no
role in response to small intestinal resection.

Secretin: No trophic effect so far demonstrated.

Prolactin: May be involved in small bowel adaptation during
lactation and may stimulate hepatic growth. The role in small
bowel adaptation has not been studied so far.

In summary, gastrin probably causes the hyperplasia seen in the
body of stomach after small bowel resection, while the hyperplasia
in the remaining small intestine may be due either to other trophic
hormones or to the loss of as-yet-unidentified inhibitory factors.

Other Gastrointestinal Disorders: The role of hormones such as growth hormone, ACTH, and prolactin, and the subtleties of disturbances of balance of the agonist and antagonist relationships between these and other peptides have not so far been explored and may be important in functional disorders such as irritable bowel syndrome and constipation. A better understanding of these factors may eventually help to explain symptoms of disordered function.

Role in Other Disease States

Diabetes Mellitus and Somatostatin: The following observations have recently been made with respect to diabetes mellitus and the respective roles of insulin, glucagon, and somatostatin.

1. Somatostatin excess can cause glucose intolerance in the presence of hypoglucagonemia and hypoinsulinemia.

2. In juvenile diabetes, somatostatin infusion causes a sustained lowering of blood glucose, reversed by infusion of physiologic quantities of glucagon, proving that the latter contributes to hyperglycemia.

3. In maturity-onset diabetes, somatostatin causes an initial modest fall in blood glucose, which is later reversed. Glucagon does not seem to contribute to hyperglycemia in this situation.

4. Glucagon is important in the development of ketoacidosis. This has been shown by somatostatin infusion, during insulin withdrawal.

5. In juvenile diabetes, the number of pancreatic D-cells is increased (Orci et al., 1976), however, the opposite is not true in maturity onset diabetes.

6. Somatostatin may have a role in treating juvenile diabetes and may reduce insulin requirement (Meissner et al., 1975; Gerich et al., 1977).

7. Microvascular complications of diabetes mellitus that are often associated with exaggerated growth hormone responses to various stimuli may be suppressed by somatostatin (Hansen et al., 1975). Changes in plasma hPP have also been described in diabetes; levels are higher in uncontrolled diabetes than in controls. PP-cell hyperplasia has been shown in juvenile-onset diabetes.

Appetite Control and Cholecystokinin (CCK): Evidence recently was presented that CCK influences appetite control (Antin et al., 1975) in rats. The satiety behavior in rats requires the presence of food in the small intestine. When chronic gastric fistulae are created in rats, so that food does not enter the small intestine, feeding continues. However, intraperitoneal injections of CCK, as large doses of gastrin, produce satiety behavior. Similar effects have been shown in rhesus monkeys. This suggests that gut hormones may influence appetite, and thus food intake.

Gastrointestinal Hormones in Chronic Renal Failure and After Renal Transplantation: Elevated motilin, hPP, GIP, and gastrin were found in fasting patients with chronic renal failure and may contribute to gastrointestinal disturbances often seen in these patients. Renal transplant recipients invariably show hyper-gastrinemia regardless of graft excretory function and graft survival time, and when peptic ulceration develops in renal transplant patients the ratio of GIP to gastrin is lower than in patients who do not have dyspepsia. This ratio may prove useful in rational prophylactic use of cimetidine in these cases (Collins et al., 1978).

Gastric Inhibitory Polypeptide and Its Glucagonotropic Action in Cirrhosis of the Liver: It has been shown that the glucagonotropic action of GIP is exhibited in this disease and that this action may be pathogenetic in glucose intolerance sometimes seen (Dupre et al., 1978) in cirrhosis.

Paralytic Ileus and Ceruletide: Ceruletide is a synthetic deca-peptide extracted from the skin of an Australian frog, and is similar to CCK-PZ and gastrin in its structure of the C-terminal portion. It causes dilatation of the cardia, gastric and pancreatic secretion, a brief pylorospasm, gallbladder contraction, and strong peristalsis of the small bowel and some peristalsis of colon. The drug has been successfully used in 58 patients with paralytic ileus where there was no response to neostigmine. Intramuscular use of the drug in postoperative cases for as long as 12 days was not accompanied by any serious side effects or tachyphylaxis (Haas and Rueft, 1978). The drug has also been used intravenously in Germany (Hartung and Waldmann, 1978).

More recently, alterations in gastrointestinal hormone levels have been shown in autonomic neuropathy, and gut hormones have been isolated from nonendocrine cancers of the lung and gastro-intestinal tract. Attempts are already being made to assay various gut hormones in per-oral biopsies of antrum, duodenum, and jejunum, and to define hormonal profiles in various disorders of the gastrointestinal tract. The future of gastrointestinal endo-crinology, therefore, looks promising in that it may increase our understanding of pathogenesis and rational treatment of many gastrointestinal as well as other disorders, and may facilitate the diagnosis of endocrine tumor syndromes by further defining their hormonal markers. At present, however, this has not been achieved, and needs a considerable amount of research and clinical effort. The diffuse endocrine system of the gut is not going to yield easily and simply to exploits of medical research and its complexities will only be unraveled at a slow but determined pace.

REFERENCES

Adamson, A.R., Grahame-Smith, D.G., Peart, W.S., and Starr, M. Pharmacological blockade of carcinoid flushing provoked by catecholamines and alcohol. *Lancet* 1969; II:293-297.

Alfidi, R.J., Bhyun, D.S., Crile, G., and Hawk, W. Arteriography and hypoglycemia. *Surg. Gynec. Obstet.* 1971; 133:447-452.

Andersson, H., Dotevall, G., Fagerberg, G., et al. Pancreatic tumor with diarrhea, hypokalemia and hypochlorhydria. *Acta Chir. Scand.* 1972; 138:102-107.

Antin, J., Gibbs, J., Holt, J., et al. Cholecystokinin elicits the complete behavioral sequence of satiety in rats. *J. Compar. Physiol. Psychia.* 1975; 89:784-790.

Arnold, R. Creutzfeldt, C., and Creutzfeldt, W. (1977): *In* V.H.T. James (Ed.), *Endocrinology, Vol. 2, Excerpta Medica.* Amsterdam, p. 440.

Balodimos, M.C., Marble, A., and Ripply, J.H. Pathological findings after long term sulfonylurea therapy. *Diabetes* 1968; 17:503-508.

Barbezat, G.O., and Grossman, M.I. Cholera like diarrhea induced by glucagon plus gastrin. *Lancet* 1971; 1:1025-1026.

Barnes, A.J., Bloom, S.R., Long, R.G., et al. New specific long acting somatostatin analogues in the treatment of pancreatic endocrine tumors. *Diabetologia* 1978; 15:217.

Becker, H.D., Reeder, D.D., and Thompson, J.C. Effect of glucagon on circulating gastrin. *Gastroenterology* 1973; 65:28-35.

Becker, W.S., Kahn, D., and Rothman, S. Cutaneous manifestations of internal malignant tumors. *Arch. Dermatol. Syphilol.* 1942; 45:1069-1080.

Blackburn, A.M., Bloom, S.R., Ebeid, F.H., and Ralphs, D.N.L. Neurotensin and the dumping syndrome. *Gut* 1978; 19:447.

Block, M.B., Roberts, ᷉.P., Kadair, R.G., et al. Multiple endocrine adenomatosis type IIb. *JAMA* 1975; 234:710-714.

Bloom, S.R., Blackburn, A.M., Besterman, H.S., et al. Measurement of neurotensin in man: A new circulating peptide hormone affecting insulin release and carbohydrate metabolism. *Diabetologia* 1978; 15:220.

Bloom, S.R., Bryant, M.G., Polak, J.M., et al. Clinic biopsies in the diagnosis of gut endocrine disorders. *Scand. J. Gastro.* 1978; 13 (supp. 49):25.

Bloom, S.R., Christofides, N.D., and Besterman, H.S. Raised motilin in diarrhea. *Gut* 1978; 19:959.

Bloom, S.R., Polak, J.M., and Pearse, A.G.E. Vasoactive intestinal peptide and watery diarrhea syndrome. *Lancet* 1973; II:14-16.

Boijsen, E., and Samuelsson, L. Angiographic diagnosis of tumors arising from the pancreatic islets. *Acta Radiol.* 1970; 10:161-175.

Bonfils, S., and Bernades, P. (1974): Zollinger Ellison syndrome: Natural history and diagnosis. *In Clinics in Gastroenterology,* Vol. 3. London: Saunders, pp. 539-557.

Broder, L.E., and Carter, S.K. Pancreatic islet cell carcinoma I—Clinical features of 52 patients. *Ann. Int. Med.* 1973; 79:101-107.

Brown, C.H., and Crile, G., Jr. Pancreatic adenoma with intractable diarrhea, hypokalemia and hypercalcemia. *JAMA* 1964; 190:30-34.

Burcharth, F., Stage, J.G., Stadil, F., Jensen, L.I., and Fisherman, K. Localization of gastrinomas by transhepatic portal catheterization and gastrin assay. *Clinics in Endocrinology and Metabolism* 1979; 8:2; 444.

Chayvialle, J.A.P., Descos, F., Bernard, C., et al. Somatostatin in mucosa of stomach and duodenum in gastroduodenal disease. *Gastroenterology* 1978; 75:13-19.

Classen, M., Gail, K., Breining, H., and Demling, L. Verner-Morrison Syndrome (Pankreatische Cholera, WDHA-syndrome). *Deutsche Med. Wochenschrift* 1972; 97:227-283.

Collins, S.M., Barnes, C.C., and Track, N.S. Gastrointestinal hormones in chronic renal failure and renal transplant recipients (1978). *Scand. J. Gastro.* 1978; 13 (suppl. 49):42.

Cowley, D., Baron, J.H., Hansley, J., and Korman, M.G. The effect of insulin hypoglycemia on serum gastrin and gastric acid in normal subjects and patients with duodenal ulcer. *Br. J. Surg.* 1973; 60:438-443.

Creutzfeldt, W. Pancreatic endocrine tumors—The riddle of their origin and hormone secretion. *Israel J. Med. Sci.* 1975; 11:762-776.

Creutzfeldt, W., Arnold, R., Creutzfeldt, C., and Track, N.S. Pathomorphological, biochemical and diagnostic aspects of gastrinomas (Zollinger Ellison Syndrome). *Human Pathology* 1975; 6:47-76.

Creutzfeldt, W., Arnold, R., Creutzfeldt, C., et al. Biochemical and morphological investigations of 30 human insulinomas. Correlation between the tumor content of insulin and proinsulin-like components and the histological and ultrastructural appearance. *Diabetologia* 1973; 9: 217-231.

Croughs, R.J.M. Glucagonoma and A-cell hyperplasia. *Clin. Gastro.* 1974; 3(3):609-620.

Croughs, R.J.M., Hulsmans, H.A.M., Israel, D.E., et al. Glucagonoma as part of the polyglandular adenoma syndrome. *Am. J. Med.* 1972; 52: 690-698.

Danforth, D.N., Triche, T., Doppman, J.L., et al. Elevated plasma proglucagon-like component with a glucagon-secreting tumor. Effect of Streptozotocin. *N. Engl. J. Med.* 1976; 295:242-245.

De Muro, P., Rownski, P., Calaresu, I., and Fragui, A. The importance of potassium in the mechanism of gastric hydrochloric acid secretion. *Acta. Med. Scand.* 1961; 170:403-410.

De Nutte, N., Somers, G., Gepts, W., et al. Pancreatic hormone release in tumor associated hypersomatostatinemia. *Diabetologia* 1978; 15:227.

Domen, R.E., Shaffer, M.B., Finke, J., et al. The glucagonoma syndrome. *Arch. Int. Med.* 1980; 140:262-263.

Dupre, J., McDonald, T.J., Caussignac, Y., and Vanvliet, S. Glucagonotropic action of gastric inhibitory polypeptide in hepatic cirrhosis. *Scand. J. Gastro.* 1978; 13 (suppl. 49):52.

Ellison, E.H., and Wilson, S.D. The Zollinger Ellison Syndrome. Reappraisal and evaluation of 260 registered cases. *Ann. Surg.* 1964; 160:512-530.

Faber, O.K., and Kehlet, H. (1979): Strategy in the diagnosis of insulinomas. *In* L. Christiansen, O. Nielsen, Stadil F. Vagn, and J.A. Stage (Eds.), *Diagnosis and Localization of Gastrointestinal Endocrine Tumors.* *Scand. J. Gastro.* 14 (suppl. 53):45-48.

Fahrenkrug, J., and Schaffalitzky de Muckadell, O.B. (1978): *VIP and Watery Diarrhea III in Gut Hormones.* S.R. Bloom (Ed.). Edinburgh, London, New York: Churchill Livingstone, pp. 576-577.

Fahrenkrug, J., and Schaffalitzky de Muckadell, O.B. (1979): Verner Morrisson Syndrome and vasoactive intestinal polypeptide. *In* L. Christiansen, O. Nielsen, Stadil F. Vagn, and J.G. Stage (Eds.), *Diagnosis and Localization of Gastrointestinal Endocrine Tumors. Scand. J. Gastroent.* 14 (suppl. 53):57-60.

Fahrenkrug, J., and Schaffalitzky de Muckadell, O.B. Radioimmunoassay of vasoactive intestinal polypeptide (VIP) in plasma. *J. Lab. Clin. Med.* 1977; 89:1379-1388.

Fajans, S.S., and Floyd, J.C., Jr. Fasting hypoglycemia in adults. *N. Engl. J. Med.* 1976; 294:766-772.

Fallucca, F., Carrata, R., Tamburrano, G., et al. Effect of caerulein and pancreozymin on insulin secretion in normal subjects and in patients with insulinoma. *Hormone Metabol. Res.* 1972; 4:55.

Farrell, R.L., Castell, D.O., and McGuigan, J.E. Measurements and comparisons of lower esophageal sphincter pressures and serum gastrin levels in patients with gastroesophageal reflux. *Gastroenterology* 1974; 67: 415-422.

Frerichs, H., and Creutzfeldt, W. Hypoglycemia. 1. Insulin secreting tumours. *Clin. Endocrinol. Metab.* 1976; 5:747-767.

Gagel, R.F., Costanza, M.E., De Lellis, R.A., et al. Streptozotocin treated Verner-Morrison syndrome. *Arch. Int. Med.* 1976; 136:1429-1435.

Ganda, O.P., Weis, G.C., Stuart Solldner, J., et al. Somatostatinoma, a-somatostatin containing tumor of the endocrine pancreas. *N. Engl. J. Med.* 1977; 296:963-967.

Geffroy, Y. (1967): *Le Syndrome Carcinoidien. Pathologie et Biologie.* 12:1149-1152.

Gerich, J.E., Lorenzi, M., Bier, D.M., et al. Effects of physiologic levels of glucagon and growth hormone on human carbohydrate and lipid metabolism. Studies involving administration of exogenous hormone with somatostatin. *J. Clin. Invest.* 1976; 75:875-884.

Gerich, J.E., Schultz, T.A., Lewis, S.B., and Karam, J.H. Clinical evaluation of somatostatin as a potential adjunct to insulin in the management of diabetes mellitus. *Diabetologia* 1977; 13(1):537-544.

Gleeson, M.H., Bloom, S.R., Polak, J.M., et al. Endocrine tumor in kidneys affecting small bowel structure, motility and absorptive function. *Gut* 1971; 12:773-782.

Grahame Smith, D.G. (1972): *The Carcinoid Syndrome.* London: Heinemann, p. 76.

Grahame Smith, D.G. Natural history and diagnosis of the carcinoid syndrome. *Clin. Gastro.* 1974; 3:3,575-594.

Gregory, R.A., and Tracy, H.J. The constitution and properties of two gastrins extracted from hog antral mucosa. *Gut* 1964; 5:103-114.

Haas, W., and Rueft, F. Clinical experience with ceruletide in the treatment of Ileus. *Scand J Gastroent.* 1978; 13 (suppl. 49):72.

Hammer, S., and Sale, G. Multiple hormone producing islet cell carcinomas of the pancreas. *Hum. Pathol.* 1975; 6:349-362.

Hansen, A.P., Christensen, S.E., and Lundbaek, K. The effect of somatostatin on the rise of growth hormone and glucagon induced by arginine and L-dopa in diabetic patients. *Scand. J. Clin. Lab. Invest.* 1975; 35: 205-210.

Hansky, J., Ho, P., Korman, M.G., and Stern, A.I. Pancreatic polypeptide release in man. Studies in ulcer disease and after gastric surgery. *Scand. J. Gastroent* 1978; 13 (suppl. 49):78.

Hansky, J., and Cain, M.D. Radioimmunoassay of gastrin in human serum. *Lancet* 1969; ii:1388-1390.

Hartung, H., and Waldmann, D. Clinical experiences with ceruletide continuous intravenous drip in the treatment of the paralytic ileus. *Scand. J. Gastro.* 1978; 13 (suppl. 49):81.

Helander, H.F. Stereological changes in rat parietal cells after vagotomy and antrectomy. *Gastroenterology* 1976; 71:1010-1018.

Holst, J.J. Gut endocrine tumor syndromes. *Clin. Endocrinol. Metab.* 1979; 8:2:413-432.

Holst, J.J. (1978): *Glucagonomas in Gut Hormones.* S.R. Bloom (Ed.). Edinburgh, New York: Churchill Livingstone, pp. 599-604.

Holst, J.J., Guldberg, O., Madsen, O., Knop, J., and Schmidt, A. The effect of intraportal and peripheral infusions of glucagon on insulin and glucose concentrations and glucose tolerance in normal man. *Diabetologia* 1977; 13:487-490.

Holst, J.J., and Ingemansson, S. Functional studies, diagnoses, treatment and control in patients with glucagonoma syndrome. *Diabetologia* 1976; 12:399.

Horton, E.W. Hypotheses on physiologic roles of prostaglandins. *Physiol. Rev.* 1969; 49:122-161.

Ingemansson, S.G. (1977): Pancreatic and intestinal vein catheterization with hormone assay. A localization procedure for gastrointestinal endocrine tumors. Bulletin No. 13, Department of Surgery, Univ. Lund, 221 85 Lund (thesis) 32 pp.

Ingemansson, S., Larsson, L.I., Lunderquist, A.K., and Stadil, F. Pancreatic vein catheterization with gastrin assay in normal patients and in patients with the Zollinger Ellison Syndrome. *Am. J. Surg.* 1977; 134:558-563.

Isenberg, J.I., Walsh, J.H., and Grossman, M.I. Zollinger Ellison Syndrome. *Gastroent.* 1973; 63:140-165.

Isenberg, J.I., Walsh, J.H., Passaro, E., Moore, E.W., and Grossman, M.I. Unusual effect of secretin on serum gastrin, serum calcium and gastric acid secretion in a patient with suspected Z-E-S. *Gastroent.* 1972; 62:626-631.

Jaffe, B.M., and Condon, S. Prostaglandins E and F in endocrine diarrheagenic syndrome. *Ann. Surg.* 1976; 184:516-524.

Jaffe, B.M., Kopen, D.F., Deschryver-Kecskemeti, K., et al. Indomethacin responsive pancreatic cholera. *N. Engl. J. Med.* 1977; 297:817-821.

Kahn, C.R., Levy, A.G., Gardner, J.D., et al. Pancreatic cholera beneficial effects of treatment with streptozotocin. *N. Engl. J. Med.* 1975; 292:941-945.

Kaneko, H., Yanaihara, N., Ito, S., et al. Somatostatinoma of the duodenum. *Cancer* 1979; 44:2273-2279.

Kaplan, E.L., Saxena, N., and Peskin, G.W. Prostaglandins a possible mediator of diarrhea in endocrine syndromes. *Surg. Forum* 1970; 21:94-95.

Kavlie, H., and White, T.T. Pancreatic islet cell tumors and hyperplasia: Experience in 14 Seattle hospitals. *Ann. Surg.* 1972; 175:326-355.

Keynes, W.M. Quoted by V. Marks and E. Samols. Insulinoma: Natural history and diagnosis. *Clin. Gastroenterol.* 1974; 3:559-573.

Kimberg, D.V., Field, M., Johnson, J., et al. Stimulation of an islet mucosal adenyl cyclase by cholera enterotoxin and prostaglandins. *J. Clin. Invest.* 1971; 50:1218-1230.

Koenen-Schamhling, B., Hartwick, G., and Dittrich, H. Verner Morrison

syndrome: A case report. *Munch. Med. Wochenschift* 1970; 112:
98-101.

Kolts, B.E., Herbst, C.A., and McGuigan, J.E.   Calcium and secretin stimulated
gastrin release in Z-E-S. *Ann. Int. Med.* 1974; 81:758-762.

Kovacs, K., Horvath, E., Ezrin, C., et al.   Immunoreactive somatostatin in
pancreatic islet-cell carcinoma accompanied by ectopic ACTH syndrome.
Lancet 1977; 1:1365-1366.

Kraft, A.R., Tompkins, R.K., Endahl, G.L., and Zollinger, R.M.   Alterations
in membrane transport produced by diarrheagenic non-beta islet cell
tumors of the pancreas. *Surg. Forum* 1969; 20:338-340.

Krejs, G.Y., Walsh, J.H., Morawski, S.G., and Fordtran, J.S.   Intractable
diarrhea.   Intestinal perfusion studies and plasma VIP concentrations
in patients with pancreatic cholera syndrome and surreptitious inges-
tion of laxatives and diuretics. *Am. J. Dig. Dis.* 1977; 22:280-292.

Lai, K.S.   Studies on gastrin. *Gut* 1964; 5:327-341.

Lambling, A., Bonfils, S., Bader, J.P., and Dubrasguet, M.   Le pouvoir
secretagogue gastrique des urines de l'homme (PSU).   Interet clinique
en particulier dans le syndrome de Zollinger-Ellison. *Gastroenterologia*
1965; 103:152-160.

Lamers, C.B.H., Stadil, F., and Van Tongeren, J.H.M.   Prevalence of endocrine
abnormalities in patients with the Zollinger Ellison Syndrome and in
their families. *Am. J. Med.* 1978; 64:607-612.

Lamers, C.B.H., and Van Tongeren, J.H.M.   Comparative study of the value
of the calcium, secretin and meal stimulated increase in serum gastrin
to the diagnosis of Z-E-S. *Gut* 1977; 18:128-134.

Larsson, L.I.   Endocrine pancreatic tumors. *Hum. Pathol.* 1978; 9:401-416.

Larsson, L.I., Rehfeld, J.F., Sundler, F., and Hakanson, R.   Pancreatic gastrin
in foetal and neonatal rats. *Nature* 1976; 262:609-610.

Larsson, L.I., Grimelius, L., Hakanson, R., et al.   Mixed endocrine pancreatic
tumors producing several peptide hormones. *Am. J. Pathol.* 1975;
79:271-284.

Larsson, L.I., Hirsch, M.A., Holst, J.S., et al.   Pancreatic somatostatinoma:
Clinical features and physiological implication. *Lancet* 1977; 1:666-
668.

Le Douarin, N.M. (1978): The embryological origin of the endocrine cells
associated with the digestive tract. *In* S.R. Bloom (Ed.), *Gut Hormones*.
Edinburgh: Churchill Livongstone, pp. 49-56.

Leupold, D., Poley, J.R., and Schlegel, W.   Multiple hormone-producing
ganglioneuroma in a child with WDHA-syndrome. *Scand. J.
Gastroent.* 1978; 13 (suppl. 49):113.

Like, A.A., and Orci, L.   Embryogenesis of the human pancreatic islets.
Diabetes 1972; 21 (suppl.):511-534.

Like, A.A., Steinke, J., Jones, E.E., and Cahill, G.F., Jr.   Pancreatic studies in
mice with spontaneous diabetes. *Am. J. Pathol.* 1965; 46:621-644.

Lipshutz, W.H., Gaskins, R.D., Lukash, W.M., and Sode, J.   Hypogastrinemia
in patients with lower esophageal sphincter incompetence.
Gastroenterology 1974; 67:423-427.

Lopes, V.M., Reis, D.D., and Cunha, A.B.   Islet cell adenoma of the pancreas
with reversible watery diarrhea and hypokalemia. *Am. J. Gastro.*
1970; 53:17-35.

Lowbeer, T.S., Harvey, R.F., and Davis, E.R.   Abnormalities of serum
cholecystokinin and gallbladder emptying in coeliac disease. *N. Engl.
J. Med.* 1975; 292:961-963.

Mallinson, C.N., Bloom, S.R., Warin, A.P., et al. A glucagonoma syndrome. *Lancet* 1974; II:1-5.

Malmstrom, J., Stadil, F., and Christensen, K.C. Effect of truncal vagotomy on gastroduodenal content of gastrin. *Br. J. Surg.* 1977; 64:34-38.

Marks, I.N., Bank, S., and Louw, J.H. Islet cell tumor of the pancreas with reversible watery diarrhea and achlorhydria. *Gastroenterology* 1967; 52:695-708.

Marks, V., and Rose, F.C. (1965): *In Hypoglycemia.* Oxford: Blackwell Scientific Publications.

Marliss, E.B., Aoki, T.T., Unger, R.H., Stuart Soeldner, J., and Cahill, G.F., Jr. Glucagon levels and metabolic effects in fasting man. *J. Clin. Invest.* 1970; 49:2256-2270.

Martini, G.A., Strohmeyer, G., Hareg, P., and Gused, W. Inselzella denom des Pankreas mit urtikarielleum, exanthem, durchfallen sowie kalium ant eiweissverlust uber den darm. *Deut. Med. Wochenschrift* 1964; 89:313-322.

Matsumoto, K.K., Peter, J.B., Raymond, G., et al. Watery diarrhea and hypokalemia associated with pancreatic islet cell adenoma. *Gastroenterology* 1966; 50:230-242.

McCrossan, M.V., Polak, J.M., Bloom, S.R., Hobbs, S., and Pearse, A.G.E. Duodenal bombesin cell pathology. *Gut* 1977; 18:A410. (abstract)

McGavran, M.H., Unger, R.H., Recant, L., et al. A glucagon secreting alpha-cell carcinoma of the pancreas. *N. Engl. J. Med.* 1966; 274: 1408-1413.

McGuigan, J.E., and Trudeau, W.L. Studies with antibodies to gastrin. *Gastroent.* 1970; 58:139-150.

Meissner, C., Thum, C., Beischer, W., et al. Antidiabetic action of somatostatin assessed by the artificial pancreas. *Diabetes* 1975; 24:988-996.

Merimee, T.J. (1977) Spontaneous hypoglycemia in man. *In* G.H. Stollerman (Ed.), *Advances in Internal Medicine.* Chicago: Yearbook Medical Publishers Inc. Vol. 22, pp. 301-317.

Miller, D.R. Functioning adenomas of pancreas with hyperinsulinism. *Arch. Surg.* 1965; 90:509-520.

Modlin, I.M., Bloom, S.R., and Mitchell, S.J. Role of VIP in diarrhea. *Gut* 1977; 18:A418.

Moertel, C.G., Dockerty, M.B., and Baggenstoss, A.H. Multiple primary malignant neoplasms I, II, and III. *Cancer* 1961; 14:221-248.

Mortimer, C.H., Carr, D., Lind, T., et al. Effects of growth hormone release inhibiting hormone on circulating glucagon, insulin and growth hormone in normal, diabetic, acromegalic and hypopituitary patients. *Lancet* 1974; 1:697-701.

Murray, J.S., Paton, R.R., and Opoe, C.E., II. Pancreatic tumor associated with flushing and diarrhea. Report of a case. *N. Engl. J. Med.* 1961; 264:436-439.

Norton, J.A., Kahn, R.K., Schiebinger, R., et al. Amino acid deficiency and the skin rash associated with glucagonoma. *Ann. Int. Med.* 1979; 91: 213-215.

Novis, B.H., Banks, S., and Marks, T.W. Exocrine pancreatic function in intestinal malabsorption and small bowel disease. *Am. J. Dig. Dis.* 1972; 17:489-494.

Oberndorfer, S. Karzinoide Tumoren des Dunndarms. Frankfurter. *Z. Pathol.* 1907; 1:426

O'Connor, F.A., McLoughlin, J.C., and Buchanan, K.D. Impaired immuno-reactive secretin release in coeliac disease. *Br. Med. J.* 1977; 1:811–812

Orci, L., Baetens, D., Rufener, C., et al. Hypertrophy and hyperplasia of somatostatin containing D cells in diabetes. *Proc. Nat. Acad. Sci. U.S.A.* 1976; 73:1338–1342.

Pabst, K., Kummerle, F., Hennekenser, H.H., and Mappes, G. Beitrag zum Krank heitshild des Verner-Morrison-syndroms. *Deut. Med. Wochenschrift* 1969; 94:9–13.

Page, S.A. Les tumeurs carcinoides: bilan provisoire et prospectives. *Biol. Med.* 1967; 56:421–453.

Passaro, E., Jr., Basso, N., and Walsh, J.H. Calcium challenge in the Zollinger Ellison Syndrome. *Surgery* 1972; 72:60–67.

Pearse, A.G.E. Neurocristopathy, neuroendocrine pathology and the APUD concept. *Z. Krebsforchung* 1975; 84:1–18.

Pedersen, N.B., Johnson, L., and Holst, J.J. Necrolytic migratory erythema and glucagon cell tumor of the pancreas: The glucagonoma syndrome. *Acta Dermat.* (Stockholm) 1976; 56:391–395.

Pictet, R.L., Rall, L.B., Phelps, P., and Rutter, W.J. The neural crest and the origin of the insulin producing and other gastrointestinal hormone producing cells. *Science* 1976; 191:191–192.

Polak, J.M., Aynsley Green, A., Bloom, S.R., and Wigglesworth, J.S. Nesidioblastosis as a cause of sudden neonatal death. *Scand. J. Gastro.* 1978; 13 (suppl. 49):143.

Polak, J.M., Bloom, S.R., McCrossan, M., et al. Abnormalities of endocrine cell in patients with duodenal ulcer and with chronic pancreatitis. *Gastroenterology* 1977; 72:822.

Polak, J.M., Pearse, A.G.E., Van Norrden, S., et al. Secretin cells in coeliac disease. *Gut* 1973; 14:870–874.

Power, L. A glucose responsive insulinoma. *JAMA* 1969; 207:893–896.

Priestley, J.T. Hyperinsulinism. *Ann. Roy. Coll. Surg.* 1962; 31:211–227.

Rask-Madsen, J., and Bukhave, K. (1979): Prostaglandins and chronic diarrhea Clinical aspects. *In* L. Christiansen, O. Vagn Nielsen, F. Stadil, and J.G. Stage (Eds.), *Diagnosis and Localization of Gastrointestinal Endocrine Tumours. Scand. J. Gastroenterol.* 14 (suppl. 53):73–78.

Rayford, P.L., Fender, H.R., Ramus, N.I., Reeder, D.D., and Thompson, J.C. (1975): Release and half life of CCK in man. *In* J.C. Thompson (Ed.), *Gastrointestinal Hormones.* Austin, London: University of Texas Press, pp. 301–318.

Rehfeld, J.F. (1979): The predominating antral gastrin and intestinal cholecystokinin in their common COOH terminal tetrapeptide amide. *In* J.F. Rehfeld and E. Amdrup (Eds.), *Gastrins and the Vagus.* London New York, Acad. Press, pp. 85–94.

Rehfeld, J.F. What is gastrin? A progress report on the heterogeneity of gastrin in serum and tissue. *Digestion* 1974; 11:397–405.

Rehfeld, J.F., and Stadil, F. Big gastrins in the Zollinger Ellison Syndrome. *Lancet* 1972; ii:1200.

Rehfeld, J.F., and Stadil, F. Gel filtration studies on immunoreactive gastrin in serum from Zollinger Ellison patients. *Gut* 1973; 14:369–373.

Rudick, J., Bonda, M., and Janowitz, H.D. Prostaglandin E: An inhibotor of electrolyte and stimulant of enzyme secretion in the pancreas. *Fed. Proc.* 1970; 29:445.

Rudo, N.D., Rosenberg, I.H., and Wissler, R.W. The effect of partial

starvation and glucagon treatment on intestinal villous morphology
and cell migration. *Proc. Sci. Exp. Biol. Med.* 1976; 152:277-280.
Said, S.I. (1978): VIP and watery diarrhea: IV. *In* S.R. Bloom (Ed.),
Gut Hormones. Edinburgh: Churchill Livingstone, pp. 578-579.
Salinas, D., Jr., Mangurten, H.H., and Roberts, S.S. Functioning islet cell
adenoma in the newborn. *Pediatrics* 1968; 41:646-653.
Sherwin, R.S., Fischer, M., Hendler, R., and Felig, P. Hyperglucogonemia
and blood glucose regulation in normal, obese and diabetic subjects.
N. Engl. J. Med. 1976; 294:455-461.
Simon, N., Warner, R.R., Baron, M.G., and Rudavsky, A.Z. Intraarterial
irradiation of carcinoid tumors of the liver. *Am. J. Roent. Radium
Ther. Nuclear Med.* 1968; 102:552-561.
Sircus, W., Brunt, P.W., Walker, R.J., et al. Two cases of "pancreatic
cholera" with features of peptide secreting adenomatosis of the
pancreas. *Gut* 1970; II:197-205.
Sive, A., Vinik, A., Vantonder, S., and Lund, A. Impaired pancreatic
polypeptide secretion in chronic pancreatitis. *J. Clin. Endoc. Metab.*
1978; 47:556-559.
Solcia, E., Capella, C., Polak, J.M., et al. Ultrastructural identification of
tumor cell types in 42 endocrine tumors of the pancreas. *Scand. J.
Gastroenterol.* 1978; 13 (suppl. 49):170.
Stadil, F., and Stage, J.G. (1979): Gastrinomas as model for duodenal ulcer
disease. *In* J.F. Rehfeld and E. Amdrup (Eds.), *Gastrin and the Vagus.*
London, New York, Academic Press.
Stadil, F., and Rehfeld, J.F. Radioimmunoassay of gastrin in human serum.
Scand. J. Gastroent. 1971; (suppl. 9):61-65.
Stage, J.G., and Stadil, F. The clinical diagnosis of the Zollinger-Ellison
Syndrome. *Scand. J. Gastroent.* 1979; 14, (suppl. 53):79-91.
Stage, J.G., Stadil, F., and Fischerman, K. (1978): New aspects in the
treatment of the Zollinger-Ellison Syndrome. *In* W. Creutzfeldt (Ed.),
Cimetidine. Amsterdam, Oxford: Excerpta Medica, pp. 137-148.
Stefanini, P., Carboni, M., and Patrassi, N. Surgical treatment and prognosis
of insulinomas. *Clin. Gastroenterol.* 1974; 3:697-709.
Stefanini, P., Carboni, M., Petrassi, N., and Basoli, A. Beta islet cell tumors
of the pancreas: Results of a statistical study on 1067 cases collected.
Surgery 1974; 75:597-609.
Stoker, D.J., and Wynn, V. Pancreatic islet cell tumor with watery diarrhea
and hypokalemia. *Gut* 1970; II:911-920.
Straus, E., and Yalow, R.S. (1975): Differential diagnosis of hypergastrinemia.
In J.C. Thompson (Ed.), *Gastrointestinal Hormones.* Austin and London,
Univ. of Texas Press, pp. 99-113.
Straus, E., and Yalow, R.S. Studies on the distribution and degradation of
heptadecapeptide, big and big big gastrins. *Gastroent.* 1974; 66:936-943.
Sturdevant, R.A., and Kun, T.L. (1974): Gastrin and gastroesophageal
sphincter competence. *In* E.E. David (Ed.), *Proc. 4th Symp. Gastro-
intestinal Motility.* Vancouver: Mitchell Press, pp. 125-130.
Sweet, R.D. A dermatosis specifically associated with a tumor of pancreatic
alpha cells. *Br. J. Dermat.* 1974; 90:301-308.
Taylor, K.W. (1972): The biosynthesis and secretion of insulin. *In* D.A.
Pyke (Ed.), *Clinics in Endocrinology and Metabolism.* Vol. I. London:
Saunders, pp. 601-622.
Tompkins, R.K., Hardacre, J.M., Tzagournis, M., and Greider, M. Definitive

diagnosis of insulin secreting tumors of the pancreas. *Surg. Gynec. Obstet.* 1967; 125:1069-1074.

Turner, R.C., and Heding, L.G. Plasma proinsulin, C-peptide and insulin in diagnostic suppression tests for insulinomas. *Diabetologia* 1977; 13: 571-577.

Turner, R.C., and Johnson, P.C. Suppression of insulin release by fish-insulin induced hypoglycemia with reference to the diagnosis of insulinomas. *Lancet* 1973; 1:1483-1485.

Turner, R.C., Oakley, N.W., and Nabarro, J.D.N. Changes in plasma insulin during ethanol induced hypoglycemia. *Metabolism* 1973; 22:111-121.

Valenzuela, J.E., Taylor, I.L., and Walsh, J.H. Pancreatic polypeptide (pp) response to a meal in pancreatitis. *Gastroenterology* 1978; 74:1149.

Verner, J.V. (1968): Clinical syndromes associated with noninsulin producing tumors of the pancreatic islets. *In* L. Demling and R. Ottenjann (Eds.), *Noninsulin Producing Tumors of the Pancreas.* Stuttgart: Georg Thieme Verlag, pp. 165-186.

Verner, J.V., and Morrison, A.B. Islet cell tumor and a syndrome of refractory watery diarrhea and hypokalemia. *Am. J. Med.* 1958; 25:374-380.

Verner, J.V., and Morrison, A.B. Endocrine pancreatic islet disease with diarrhea. Report of a case due to diffuse hyperplasia of non B islet tissue with a review of 54 additional cases. *Arch. Int. Med.* 1974; 133:492-500.

Walsh, J. (1979): Pathogenetic role of the gastrins. *In* J.F. Rehfeld and E. Amdrup (Eds.), *Gastrins and the Vagus.* London and New York: Academic Press.

Welbourn, R.B., Polak, J.M., Bloom, S.R., et al. (1978): Apudomas of the pancreas. *In* S.R. Bloom (Ed.), *Gut Hormones.* Edinburgh: Churchill Livingstone, pp. 561-569.

Wilder, R.M., Allan, F.N., Power, M.H., and Robertson, H.E. Carcinoma of islands of pancreas: Hyperinsulinism and hypoglycemia. *JAMA* 1927; 89:348-355.

Wilkinson, D.S. Necrolytic migratory erythema with carcinoma of the pancreas. *Trans. St. John's Hosp. Dermatol. Soc.* 1973; 59:244-250.

Willems, G., Van Steenkiste, Y., and Limbosch, J.M. Stimulating effects of gastrin on cell proliferation kinetics in the canine fundic mucosa. *Gastroenterology* 1972; 62:583-589.

Yalow, R.S., and Berson, S.A. And now 'big, big' gastrin. *Biochem. Biophys. Res. Comm.* 1972; 48:391-394.

Yalow, R.S., and Berson, S.A. Radioimmunoassay of gastrins. *Gastroent.* 1970; 58:1-14.

Zenker, R., Forrell, M.M., and Erpenbeck, R. Zur Kenntnis eines seltenen durch ein Pankreasadenom Verusachten Krankheitssyndroms. *Deut. Wochenschrift* 1966; 91:634-638.

Zollinger, R.M., and Coleman, D.W. (1974): *In Influence of Pancreatic Tumors on the Stomach.* Springfield: Charles C. Thomas.

Zollinger, R.M., Tompkins, R.K., Amerson, J.R., et al. Identification of the diarrhoegenic hormone associated with non-beta islet-cell tumors of the pancreas. *Ann. Surg.* 1968; 168:502-521.

Zollinger, R.M., and Ellison, E.H. Primary peptic ulcerations of the jejunum associated with islet cell tumors of the pancreas. *Ann. Surg.* 1955; 142:709-723.

4

Perinatal Hypothyroidism and Brain Function

WALTER B. ESSMAN

Alterations in fetal and perinatal thyroid functions can exert significant influences upon the morphologic, biochemical, and functional integrity of the mammalian brain. The bases of early thyroid dysfunction, though varied, depending upon maternal factors, endogenous hormone and/or metabolic influences, mechanical or toxic effects, etc., ultimately affect the same general tissue parameters. In general, these may be said to concern tissue growth and development, protein synthesis and nitrogen metabolism, oxygen consumption and thermogenesis, ion transport across cell membranes, the structure and function of mitochondria, the synthesis of proteins and nucleic acids, enzyme activity, and the metabolism of several biogenic amines. Such tissue effects of the thyroid hormones, 1-thyroxine and 1-triiodothyronine, are reflected in the early postnatal disposition of peripheral as well as central nervous system tissue.

The feedback system between the thyroid hormones and the pituitary can be permanently altered by even brief episodes of hypothyroidism during the perinatal period (Bakke et al., 1970). In rats, where the development of the hypothalamic regulatory mechanisms for thermogenesis is dependent upon thyroxine secretion, there is an impairment in the development of such regulation processes in hypothyroidism (Hamburgh, 1968). The maturation of both the pituitary and hypothalamic feedback systems with the thyroid can be compromised by fetal or perinatal

hypothyroidism. The deficit in neurologic function attending neonatal hypothyroidism has been well recognized, and has included
a spectrum of defects from deaf mutism and intellectual dysfunction to impaired somatic growth (Querido and Swaab, 1975).
Fetal thyroid hormone deficiency has accounted for a wide range
of neurochemical defects in the monkey during development
(Holt et al., 1975). A reduced brain cell size in the monkey
cerebrum and cerebellum was suggested by the reduced levels of
protein, RNA, cholesterol, K, Na-ATPase, and carbonic anhydrase.
It is not surprising, therefore, that structural, functional, and
chemical changes in the developing nervous system result from fetal
and perinatal thyroid deficiency.

One animal model that has been particularly appropriate for
the investigation of fetal hypothyroidism is the rat. In this species
the effects of fetal thyroidectomy have produced rather consistent
morphologic alterations, including poorly developed and dispersed
cells in the cerebral cortex (Eayrs, 1955), reduced dendritic growth
and arborization, and a marked impairment of cerebellar synaptic
development (Nicholson and Altman, 1972). Hypothyroidism has
a rather marked effect on the capillary density of the cerebral
cortex (Eayrs, 1954), where such a reduction in the microvascula-
ture could account for a reduction in the availability of substrate
for a number of critical metabolic events in the developing nervous
system.

Another animal that provides an interesting model for brain
changes with fetal hypothyroidism is the sheep, which usually has
a 150-day gestation period. In sheep where hypothyroidism
resulted from thyroidectomy at 90 to 110 days of gestation,
delayed myelination and retarded cell growth were noted
(Erenberg et al., 1974). Significantly reduced cerebral cortical
weight occurred when fetal sheep were thyroidectomized at 50
to 60 days of gestation (McIntosh et al., 1979a). Cytoarchitectural
studies of the cerebellum from sheep thyroidectomized at 56 to
96 days of gestation revealed fragmentation of myelin, a paucity
of intracytoplasmic vesicles, and a reduction in the apparently
intact synaptic junctions (Hollingsworth et al., 1975). If the fetal
sheep thyroid was removed when it began to function, at 50 to
60 days of gestational age (Barnes et al., 1957), and then pregnancy was allowed to continue to term, or before, several effects
upon brain development were observed (McIntosh et al., 1979a).
Total brain weight for thyroidectomized lambs born after 120 days
of gestation was reduced by 11.7%, and those born at term by
24.5%. The greatest weight change occurred for the cerebellum of
120-day gestational lambs (23%), although those hypothyroid

lambs born at term showed reduced tissue weight in the cerebral hemispheres (31.8%), brain stem (23.4%), and spinal cord (26.6%). An increase in the weight of the pituitary (48.1%) resulted from fetal thyroidectomy. Cystic brain cavities were also noted among some of the neonatal lambs.

There have been some biochemical studies in the brain of hypothyroid sheep, the results of which have largely conformed the more basic morphologic data. In sheep that were thyroidec- tomized at 90 to 110 days of gestation, cerebellar protein concen- tration was reduced and in cerebral tissues there was a lowered lipid concentration and an increase in C-18 fatty acids (Erenberg et al., 1974). With earlier fetal thyroidectomy (50 to 60 days of gestation) the effects of hypothyroidism appeared to be more deleterious as fetal age progressed to term (McIntosh et al., 1979b). At term, but not at 120 or 90 days of gestation, significant reductions were observed in DNA (40.1%) and protein (44.5%) content of the cerebral hemispheres, protein content of the total brain (44.1%) and spinal cord (27%), and RNA content of the total brain (37.4%). In term hypothyroid sheep there was also a reduced level of cholesterol that was most marked in the cerebellum (40.6%) and brain stem (40.5%). In several other recent studies more dynamic aspects of cellular metabolic and chemical functions in the neonatal hypothyroid sheep brain have been considered. In twin sheep, one member of which was thyroidectomized at 60 days of gestation and both members were delivered by cesearian section at 110 days of gestation, several functional aspects of neural activity were studied (Figure 1).

The synaptosomal uptake of dopamine was significantly lower in the hypothalamus ($p<0.01$) and cerebellar cortex ($p<0.01$) of euthyroid sheep brain than for the cerebral cortex, and there was no effect of hypothyroidism upon cortical dopamine uptake (Figure 2). In contrast, dopamine uptake was significantly in- creased in synaptosomes from the hypothalamus (80%; $p<0.01$) and the cerebellar cortex (130%; $p<0.01$) of hypothyroid sheep.

Highly significant decreases in norepinephrine uptake by cortical synaptosomes ($p<0.001$) were observed (Figure 3), whereas nerve endings from the hypothalamus and cerebellar cortex did not show altered norepinephrine uptake in the tissue from hypothyroid sheep.

Serotonin (5-HT) uptake by synaptosomes from hypothyroid sheep cortex and hypothalamus was significantly reduced (250%; $p<$ 0.01, and 109%; $p<0.01$, respectively); no effect of hypothyroidism was apparent upon cerebellar synaptosomal 5-HT uptake (Figure 4).

In Figure 5 the regional synaptosomal uptake of GABA has been summarized. Hypothyroidism accounted for significantly

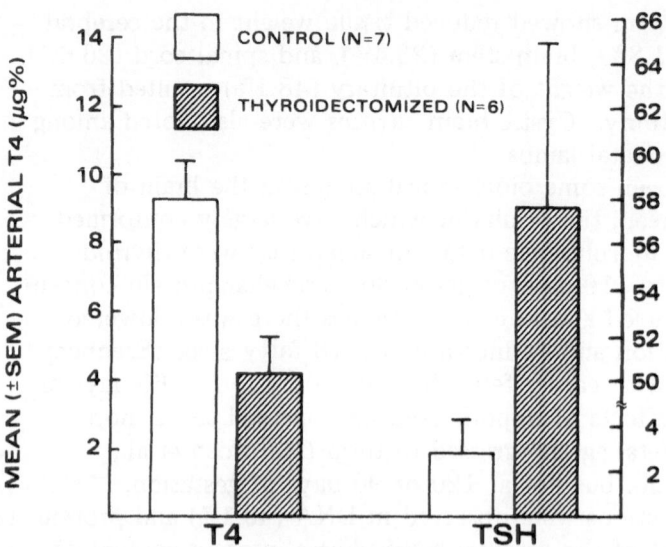

Fig. 1. Arterial T4 and Plasma TSH Levels in Control and Thyroidectomized
Neonatal Sheep

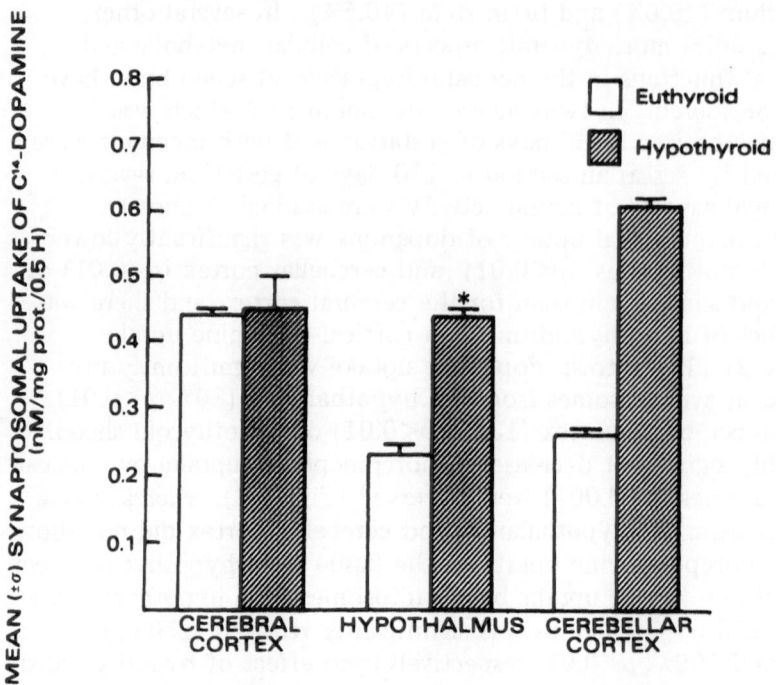

Fig. 2. Regional Synaptosomal Dopamine Uptake: Effect of Perinatal
Hypothyroidism

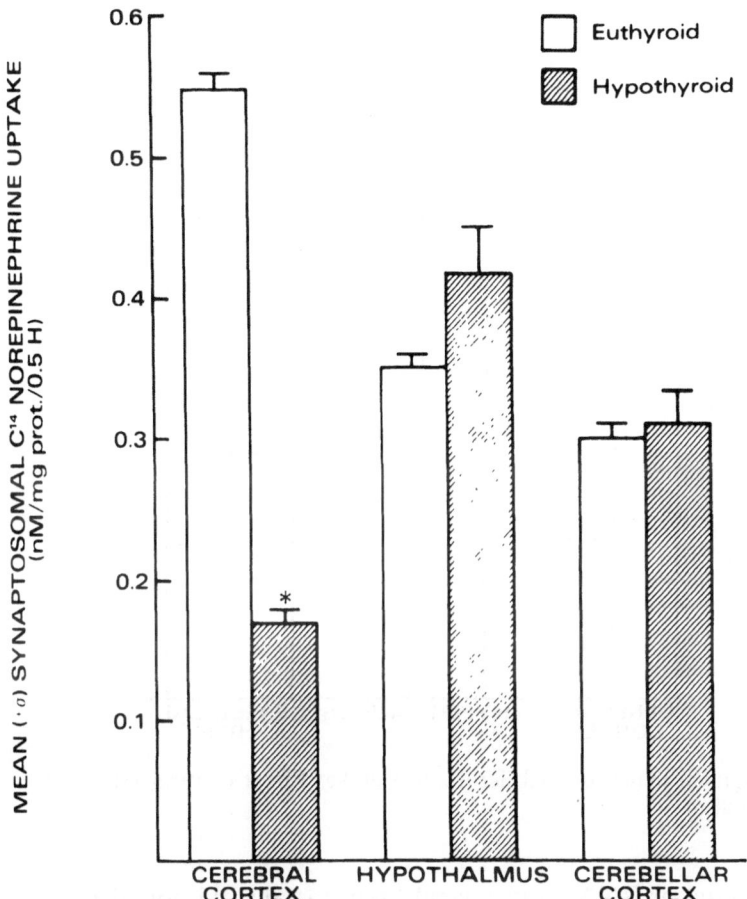

Fig. 3. Regional Synaptosomal Norepinephrine Uptake: Effect of Perinatal Hypothyroidism

increased uptake by endings from the cerebral cortex (133%; $p < 0.01$) and hypothalamus (101%; $p < 0.01$). No significant change in GABA uptake occurred for endings of the cerebellar cortex from hypothyroid sheep.

The synaptosomal uptake of histamine was significantly increased in endings from all three brain regions of the hypothyroid sheep brain (177%; $p < 0.01$; 129%; $p < 0.01$; and 111%; $p < 0.01$; respectively, for cortex, hypothalamus, and cerebellum). These are summarized in Figure 6 (Essman et al., 1979).

Several indices of neuronal function were assessed in neonatal sheep that were thyroidectomized at 64 days of gestational age. RNA synthesis measured by the rate of C^{14} orotic acid incorpora-

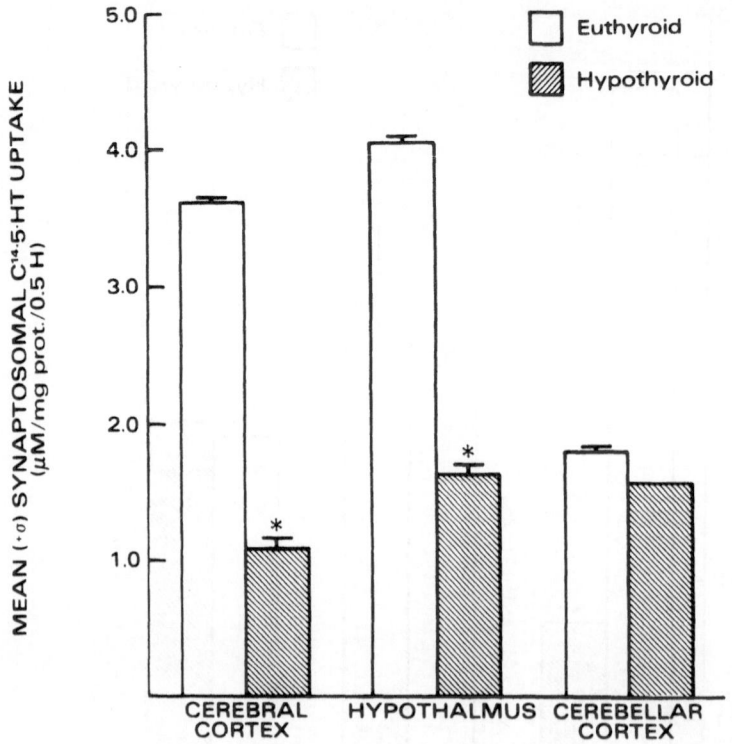

Fig. 4. Regional Synaptosomal Serotonin Uptake: Effect of Perinatal
Hypothyroidism

tion into nuclear RNA from several brain regions did not differ
for the cerebral cortex of hypothyroid (T4=4.1 ± 1.2; TSH=37.5
± 10.1) as compared with euthyroid (T4=9.2 ± 1.4; TSH=3.1 ±
1.2) neonates; mitochondrial RNA synthesis was significantly
reduced in the thalamus and hypothalamus (12%; $p<0.02$) and in
the cerebellar cortex (18%; $p<0.01$) of hypothyroid animals
(Table 1). Protein synthesis, measured by incorporation of C^{14}
leucine into synaptosomal proteins, was significantly reduced in
the hypothyroid neonates; in presynaptic nerve endings from the
cerebral cortex (32%; $p<0.01$), thalamus and hypothalamus (17%;
$p<0.02$) and cerebellar cortex (53%; $p<0.01$) protein synthesis was
reduced (Table 2). The cellular and synaptic changes attending
perinatal hypothyroidism are reflected in regional changes in the
synthesis of macromolecules relevant to effective cerebral functions
(Essman et al., 1981).
    The fetal sheep, perhaps like the monkey, for which there have
been even fewer morphologic and almost no biochemical studies in

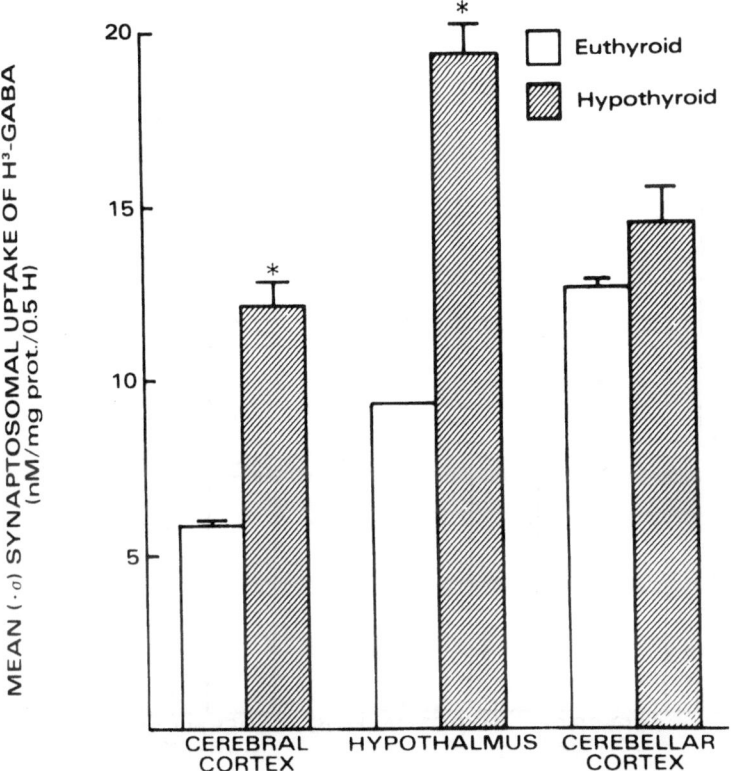

Fig. 5. Regional Synaptosomal GABA Uptake: Effect of Perinatal Hypothyroidism

the hypothyroid state, represents an excellent model by which to approximate human fetal and perinatal thyroid function in regard to brain development. There is a similar chronologic relationship between thyroid and brain development (Erenberg and Fisher, 1972; Thorburn and Hopkins, 1972); also, an autonomous fetal thyroid-pituitary axis, and the placenta is relatively impermeable to the thyroid hormones (Fisher et al., 1977).

The majority of studies concerning the morphologic, biochemical, and functional properties of postnatal brain as affected by hypothyroidism have been conducted in the rat, where early postnatal development bears some relationship to late human prenatal development (Balazs, 1972). A considerable number of studies have been carried out in the rat, demonstrating that brain tissue weight and cell size are reduced if hypothyroidism intervened during fetal or early postnatal development. Some of the earlier studies utilized postnatal methylthiouracil to effect hypothyroid-

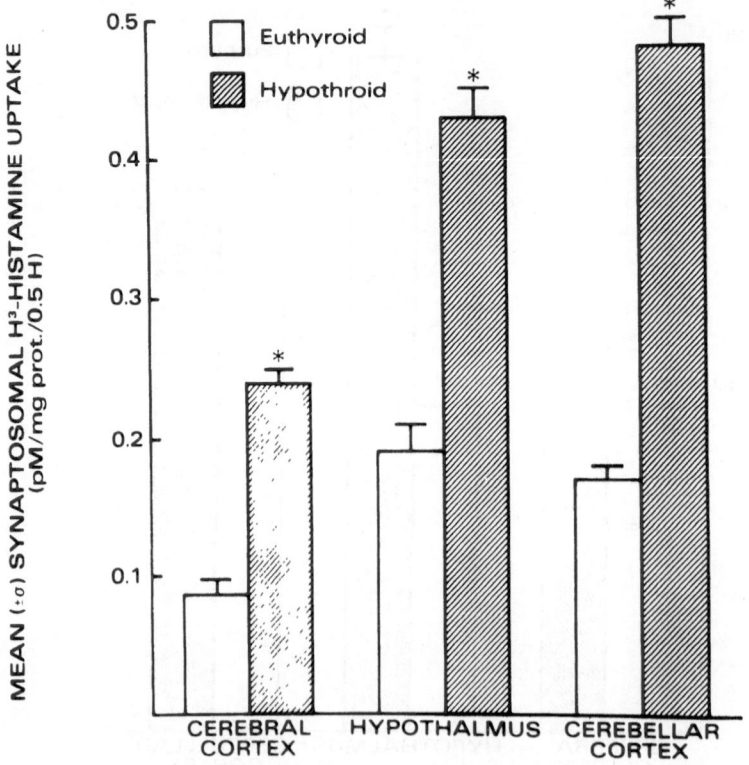

Fig. 6. Regional Synaptosomal Histamine Uptake: Effect of Perinatal
Hypothyroidism

ism and reduced brain weight (Eayrs and Taylor, 1951) was confirmed through the use of radioactive iodine in later studies
(Eayrs and Horn, 1955), where essentially the same effects were
produced. In the cerebellum of hypothyroid rats the Purkinje
cell orientation and basket cell number were reduced (Legrand,
1965), whereas glia in the cerebellum were increased (Nicholson
and Altman, 1972; Pesetsky, 1973; Clos and Legrand, 1973).
The necessity for appropriate thyroid hormone concentration for
the development, at normal rates, of postnatal parallel fiber
growth in the cerebellum has been emphasized (Lauder, 1978).
The parallel fiber is a T-shaped granule cell axon that is generated
during the second postnatal week in the rat. In 12-day-old hypothyroid rats there was increased (31%) width of the subproliferative
zone of the external granular layer during the period of granule
cell migration; the transit time of labeled cell movements to the
internal granular layer was increased by hypothyroidism, but the
rate of cell movements was decreased. Therefore, both decreased

Table 1. Mean ($\pm\sigma$) Rate of C^{14}-Orotic Acid Incorporation
(nMoles/mg Protein) Into Regional Ribonucleic Acid in Neonatal Sheep Brain

Condition	Brain Region		
	Cerebral Cortex	*Cerebellar Cortex*	*Thalamus and Hypothalamus*
Control	0.799	2.229	2.175
	(0.089)	(0.068)	(0.276)
Thyroidectomized	1.314	1.824*	1.904*
	(0.068)	(0.097)	(0.073)

*$p < .02$

cerebellar granule cell migration and parallel fiber development
accompany neonatal hypothyroidism (Lauder, 1979). An analysis
of cerebellar tissue in propylthiouracil-induced hypothyroidism in
neonatal rats revealed some thinning of the molecular layer. In
90-day-old rats, selective staining of the synaptic apparatus revealed
only 60% of the synapses visualized in euthyroid controls
(Schalock, 1977).

The development of synapses in several regions of the rat brain
implies not only the morphologic but also the biochemical integrity
of the communication network between neurons. The effects of
neonatal hypothyroidism upon synaptogenesis have been shown for
the motor and visual areas of the cerebral cortex (Cragg, 1967) and
in the molecular layer of the cerebellar cortex (Nicholson and
Altman, 1972). Biochemical studies of the synaptic region of the
rat cerebrum and cerebellum have been carried out using isolated
presynaptic nerve ending (synaptosome) preparations (Verity et al.,
1976) and a number of highly relevant findings for neonatal hypo-
thyroidosm have emerged. In cerebellar synaptosomes from hypothyroid rats there was a retardation of LDH and cytochrome C
oxidase activities and at 8 and 14 days postpartum there was a
significant reduction in protein synthesis. Increased synaptosomal
protein synthesis occurred in the cerebral cortex of hypothyroid
rats at 14, 20, and 30 days of age.

Neonatal hypothyroidism in the rat has also been shown to affect
other enzyme systems regulating substrate functions during early
development, for example, the ketone body-metabolizing enzymes.
Since pyruvate and ketone body oxidation in the developing brain
represent important bases for energy, any possible compromise in
such enzyme systems could provide for growth defects and retardation syndromes. The ketone body-metabolizing enzymes, 3-
hydroxybutyrate dehydrogenase, 3-oxoacid CoA-transferase, and
acetoacetyl CoA-thiolase, were studied for their postnatal develop-

Table 2. Mean ($\pm\sigma$) Rate of C^{14}-Leucine Incorporation
(nMoles/mg Protein/Hour)
Into Regional Synaptosomes from Neonatal Sheep Brain

| | Brain Region | | |
| | Cerebral Cortex | Cerebellar Cortex | Thalamus and Hypothalamus |
Condition			
Control	18.039 (0.078)	25.072 (1.395)	23.725 (0.304)
Thyroidectomized	12.472* (0.010)	11.093+ (0.448)	19.593* (0.800)

*$p<.02$
+$p<.01$

ment in the neonatal hypothyroid rat brain (Patel, 1979). The postnatal development of these enzymes was markedly retarded during the first four postnatal weeks. Unlike euthyroid controls, there was no decreased enzyme activity in the hypothyroid rat brain during the immediate postweaning period. For 4-week-old hypothyroid rats, both the synaptic and the nonsynaptic mitochondria showed a highly significant reduction in ketone body-metabolizing enzymes.

Enzyme synthesis by the hypothalamus has also been assessed at different stages of gestation in thyroidectomized pregnant rat (Goswami et al., 1980). Acid phosphatase activity was reduced in rats thyroidectomized on the eighth and tenth day of pregnancy, whereas alkaline phosphatase activity was higher for rats thyroidectomized on the sixth and eighth day of pregnancy. Glutamate pyruvate transaminases were significantly elevated for rats thyroidectomized on the sixth and tenth day of pregnancy. The regulatory functions of the hypothalamus, particularly as it applies to release factors and pituitary regulation, are dependent upon enzymatic regulation of energy processes for membrane transport and secretory functions, as well as relating to interactions between TRH and other releasing factors originating in the hypothalamus. For example, in neonatal hypothyroid rats the total content of TRH in the hypothalamus was slightly decreased, but the specific concentration of this peptide in the brain was increased (Oliver et al., 1980). This could be accounted for by the effect of neonatal hypothyroidism upon hypothalamic enzyme activity, such as reduced TRH synthetase (Reichlin and Mitnick, 1973) or by reduced dendritic and/or synaptic formation and input in hypothyroidism (Balazs et al., 1968; Cragg, 1970). The direct effects of TRH have also been demonstrated upon thyroid peroxidase activity, which is stimulated in the teleost fish (Bhattacharya et al., 1979).

There is evidence for TRH receptor sites in the sheep thyroid (Essman et al., 1980). These findings could point to a role for hypothalamic factors regulating TRH release that are modified in the hypothyroid state. The pituitary-thyroid system of offspring from hypothyroid mothers is activated during late gestation (Hendrich et al., 1979). Another cause of perinatal hypothyroidism in the rat is the neonatal administration of monosodium glutamate (Nemeroff et al., 1978). Whereas serum levels of the thyroid hormones are reduced, hypothalamic levels of TRH are unchanged.

Thyroid regulation of brain monoamine oxidase (MAO) activity appears a particularly relevant aspect of the relationship between thyroid hormones and their deficiency in amine substrates for this enzyme system. In the adult MAO activity is regulated by thyroxine (Spinks and Burn, 1952; Moonat et al., 1975). In 5-day-old rat fetuses from mothers treated with PTU, brain MAO activity was significantly reduced (35%), independently from brain protein content (Gripois and Fernandez, 1977). In comparison with the effects of postnatal PTU-induced hypothyroidism and MAO activity, where treatment must be extended over two weeks to produce effects (Gripois and Fernandez, 1976), it appears that MAO activity is more vulnerable to thyroxine deficiency during fetal life in the rat. Since MAO activity in the brain may be selective in its specificity for certain substrates and therefore has been characterized in at least two forms (A and B), it is possible that age differences in the development of such isozymes or differences in dependence upon thyroxine could account for the effects of fetal or postnatal hypothyroidism.

It is perhaps relevant that some consideration be given to some of the amines that represent substrates for the amine oxidases and to what extent their disposition in the brain has been affected by hypothyroidism. The whole brain pattern of norepinephrine level has been shown to be disrupted in neonatal hypothyroidism (Rastogi and Singhal, 1974, 1976), and in more detailed regional studies (Rastogi and Singhal, 1979) hypothalamic, medullary-pontine, and striatal norepinephrine levels were reduced at 30 days of age in rats rendered neonatally hypothyroid. Cerebellar NE levels were unaffected, but striatal tyrosine hydroxylase activity was markedly reduced by hypothyroidism. Dopamine levels were reduced in the striatum of hypothyroid rats, and the DA metabolite DOPAC, was reduced by 40% in the striatum. It is of interest to contrast the consequences of postnatal hypothyroidism upon the catecholamine catabolizing enzyme, MAO, in this study, with the effects of fetal hypothyroidism previously discussed. MAO activity at 30 days-of-age for rats made neonatally hypothyroid was elevated in the midbrain (14%) and decreased in the hypothalamus

(14%). Other brain regions, such as the cerebral cortex, brain
stem, and striatum, were essentially unaffected by hypothyroidism
initiated at birth. In contrast, the methylating enzyme, catechol-
O-methyl-transferase, showed increased activity in 30-day-old hypothyroid rats—in the brain stem (26%), striatum (22%), and midbrain (19%), while for the hypothalamus its activity was decreased
by 40%. The implications of these findings for catecholaminergic
synaptic dysfunction in neonatal hypothyroidism may perhaps be
appropriate for the neonatal and perinatal central nervous system,
particularly in view of related findings of decreased brain norepinephrine turnover in hypothyroidism (Jacoby et al., 1975) and
suggested alterations in noradrenergic receptor sensitivity in hypothyroidism (Emlen et al., 1972). Both pre- and postsynaptic
noradrenergic receptor mechanisms have been studied in young
PTU-induced hypothyroid rats (Gross et al., 1980). β-adrenergic
receptor functions were impaired in the cerebral cortex of hypothyroid rats, but presynaptic α-adrenergic receptors were unaffected.

   Several studies have examined the relationship between neonatal
hypothyroidism in the rat and its effects upon the brain serotoninergic system. Effects of neonatal hypothyroidism on whole brain
serotonin and its synthesizing enzyme, tryptophan hydroxylase,
were reflected in a retarded developmental pattern (Singhal et al.,
1975). In consideration of the more regionally specific brain effects
of neonatal hypothyroidism on serotoninergic neurons (Rastogi
and Singhal, 1978) in 30-day-old rats made hypothyroid at birth,
several defects were observed. A significant decrease (24%) in
tryptophan hydroxylase activity occurred, with no appreciable
change in brain tryptophan content. Decreased serotonin levels
were noted in the striatum, midbrain, and cerebellum; however,
in the pons-medulla, serotonin levels were increased by 29% in
the hypothyroid animals. The serotonin metabolite, 5-
hydroxyindoleacetic acid (5-HIAA), was increased in the striatum
(36%), midbrain (27%), and cerebellum (41%), whereas in the
hypothalamus there was a slight (16%) nonsignificant decrease.
Replacement therapy with T3 for 30 days, beginning at day 5,
reversed all of the observed changes in serotonin metabolism. It
may be appropriate, in the present context, to note that neonatal
hypothyroidism in the rat and its effect upon brain serotonin
content and metabolism can be related to an adverse relationship in
the adult animal; namely, the inhibition of brain serotonin synthesis can cause a significant decrease in T3 levels as well as a
decrease in TSH, with the latter effect probably being secondary to
a direct effect upon hypothalamic serotonin (Shopsin et al., 1974).
It is of interest that hypothyroidism-induced decrements in sero-

tonin level, and concomitant effects upon both the thyroid and hypothalamic pituitary axis, provide a basis for a continuing cycle of central effect—central regulation dynamics based upon thyroid hormone—serotonin—thyroid hormone—hypothalamic-pituitary interactions. Such dynamics certainly bear further investigation and may be particularly appropriate to a later consideration in this chapter: the issue of endemic hypothyroidism and brain function. This issue could relate, interestingly, to the question of tryptophan mediation of brain serotonin content and hence availability for thyroid regulation of T3 secretion and/or hypothalamic regulation of pituitary TSH release.

Another biogenic amine active for both neurons and mast cells in the rat brain is histamine; the mast cells of the adult thyroid gland are degranulated by the action of thyroid hormones. In the neonatal thyroidectomized rat the brain mast cell histamine was increased, by 5 days of age, to 40% above control levels (Blanco et al., 1978). The influence of thyroid hormones upon mast cell maturation would be suggested as depending upon an inhibitory control, at least in the neonatal rat; where such control is removed by neonatal thyroidectomy, histamine levels accrue. This effect might depend upon negative feedback of the reduced thyroid hormone level upon TSH, and its stimulation of adjacent mast cells, or other possible mechanisms that remain to be elucidated.

An obvious, but perhaps little explored, area of investigation in the perinatally hypothyroid state is the effect of such thyroid hormone reduction upon brain receptors. A developmental defect as reflected in brain β-adrenergic receptor sites, has been shown for neonatal hypothyroid rats (Smith et al., 1980). Muscarinic cholinergic receptors were measured in neonatal rat brain over a 6- to 35-day-of-age period after hypothyroidism initiated at birth, and did not show an appreciable change in density; in the cerebellum, however, normal age-related decrements in muscarinic cholinergic receptor density were retarded in hypothyroid animals (Patel et al., 1980). By 35 days of age receptor density in the cerebellum of hypothyroid rats was 40% greater than euthyroid controls. The age-related increment in cerebellar GABA receptors was attenuated in thyroid deficient animals. The developing neurotransmitter system receptors in the brain can therefore be profoundly influenced by thyroid status during the perinatal period. This appears particularly appropriate to several such receptor systems in the cerebellum—a site where postnatal changes in other developing morphologic and chemical systems appear to be vividly reflected.

The lipid composition of membranes that constitute some of the receptor sites in the brain for neurotransmitters, and their agonists and antagonists, seems particularly appropriate to the findings that receptor density for specific neurotransmitters can be altered by the thyroid state. There are some data to suggest that some brain lipids such as sulfatide, cerebroside, and cholesterol are reduced in neonatal hypothyroidism (Walravens and Chase, 1969), where sulfatide synthesis and cerebroside synthesis (Mantzos et al., 1973) were reduced. Myelin and synaptosomal sulfatide levels were reduced in 20- to 21-day-old rats rendered neonatally hypothyroid. Furthermore, sulfatide synthesis in myelin, mitochondria, microsomes, and synaptosomes was reduced. Hypothyroidism initiated at 30 days of age did not produce such effects, suggesting a greater neonatal susceptibility to the effects of hypothyroidism on neural membrane and meylin sulfatides (Harris and Loh, 1979). Whether such effects are reversible with thyroid hormone replacement remains to be explored.

The effects of perinatal hypothyroidism upon several parameters of brain function have been examined for the three species that have served as putative models for such dysfunction and pathology in humans. The spectrum of neurologic, behavioral, and social disorder that may occur with human thyroid disturbance is particularly relevant to the clinical perspective of this review. In that context it may be possible to make a distinction between the disorder associated with disturbed availability of thyroid hormone, or myxedematous cretinism, and the defects seen with iodine deficiency and apparently normal levels of thyroid hormones, or neurologic cretinism. There are a number of distinguishing features for each of these and perhaps the best, if not the only, available source for the study of such neurodevelopmental defects in humans has been to rely upon the data concerned with endemic goiter and endemic cretinism.

It might be initially appropriate, however, to comment upon iodine deficiency and its neurodevelopmental sequalae. While a mild to moderate deficiency can be associated with endemic goiter, a more severe endemic deficiency state can account for cretinism, usually in the absence of frank hypothyroidism. Of the cases of endemic cretinism, two distinct varieties have been identified and confirmed in several endemic regions (Hetzel, 1972). These have been termed the *myxedematous* type. In one series from the Idjivi Island in Zaire, the myxedematous form occurred in the majority of cases (Delange et al., 1972). In other major series (Lobo et al., 1963; Patel et al., 1963; Goslings et al., 1977) the neurologic form was most frequently observed. Unlike the myxedematous cretin, in the neurologic form there are no clinical signs of hypothyroidism; there is little, if any, growth retardation; and thyroid hormones do not alter the clinical presentation. Both forms exhibit pronounced intellectual retardation, but motor defects and deaf mutism are found only in the neurologic version.

The neuroanatomical and neurochemical substrates for the neurologic and behavioral impairment attending neonatal endemic cretinism, particularly of the neurologic form, have not been elucidated. However, there are studies that certainly suggest that fetal hypothyroidism is a characteristic of both types of cretinism (Dumont et al., 1969). Why this state should persist into perinatal life in the myxedatous cretin, and revert to relatively normal thyroid function in the neurologic form, may depend on the effect of the iodine deficiency upon the thyroid hormones and the tests by which thyroid hormone activity have been assessed in these states. With severe iodine deficiency there is a preferential synthesis and release of T3 over T4 (Delange et al., 1972; Koutras et al., 1970). It is therefore possible that this postnatal effect, which is reversible with iodine replacement, averts the neurologic defects seen in the myxedematous form, and can account for reasonably normal total thyroid hormone levels seen in the neurologic form. It is clear, however, that fetal hypothyroidism, common to both forms of endemic cretinism, plays an important role in the etiology of central nervous system-related defects that occur with fetal deficiency of thyroid hormones.

REFERENCES

Bakke, L.J., Gellert, R.J., and Laurence, N. The persistent effects of perinatal hypothyroidism on pituitary, thyroid, and gonadel functions. *J. Lab. Clin. Med.* 1970; 76:25-33.

Balazs, R. Effects of hormones and nutrition on brain development. *Adv. Exper. Med. Biol.* 1972; 30:385-415.

Balazs, R., Kovacs, S., Teichgraber, P., Cocks, W.A., and Eayrs, J.T. Biochemical effects of thyroid deficiency on the developing brain. *J. Neurochem.* 1968; 15:1335-1349.

Barnes, C.M., Warner, D.E., Marks, S., and Bustad, L.K. Thyroid function in fetal sheep. *Endocrinology* 1957; 60:325-327.

Bhattacharya, S., Mukherjee, D., and Sen, S. Role of synthetic mammalian thyrotropin releasing hormone on fish thyroid peroxidase activity. *Indian J. Exp. Biol.* 1979; 17:1041-1043.

Blanco, I., Rodergas, E., Picatoste, F., Sabria, J., and Garcia, A. Effect of experimental hyper- and hypothyroidism on neonatal rat brain histamine levels. *Agetns Actions* 1978; 8:384.

Clos, J., and Legrand, J. Effects of thyroid deficiency on different cell populations of the cerebellum of the young rat. *Brain Res.* 1973; 63:450-455.

Cragg, B.G. The density of synapses and neurons in the motor and visual areas of the cerebral cortex. *J. Anat.* (London) 1967; 101:639-654.

Cragg, B.G. Synapses and membranous bodies in experimental hypothyroidism. *Brain Res.* 1970; 18:297-307.

Delange, F., Camus, M., and Ermans, A.M. Circulating thyroid hormones in endemic goiter. *J. Clin. Endocrinol. Metab.* 1972; 26:149-173.

Dumont, J.E., Delange, F., and Ermans, A.M. (1969): *In* J.B. Stanbury (Ed.), *Endemic Goitre.* Washington, D.C.: Pan American Health Organization Scientific Pub. no. 193, p. 9.

Eayrs, J.T. The vascularity of the cerebral cortex in normal and cretinous rats. *J. Anat.* 1954; 88:164-173.

Eayrs, J.T. The cerebral cortex of normal and hypothyroid rats. *Acta Anat.* 1955; 25:160-183.

Eayrs, J.T., and Horn, G. The development of cerebral cortex in hypothyroid and starved rats. *Anatom. Res.* 1955; 121:53-79.

Eayrs, J.T., and Taylor, S.H. The effect of thyroid deficiency induced by methyl thiouracil on the maturation of the central nervous system. *J. Anat.* 1941; 85:350-358.

Emlen, W., Segal, D.S., and Mandell, A.J. Thyroid state: Effects on pre- and postsynaptic central noradrenergic mechanisms. *Science* 1972; 175: 79-82.

Erenberg, A., and Fisher, D.A. (1972): Thyroid hormone metabolism in the foetus. *In Foetal and Neonatal Physiology; Proc. Sir Joseph Barcroft Symposium.* Cambridge, England: Cambridge University Press, pp. 508-526.

Erenberg, A., Omori, K., Menkes, J.H., Oh, W., and Fisher, D.A. Growth and development of the thyroidectomized ovine fetus. *Pediat. Res.* 1974; 8:783-789.

Essman, E.J., Ayromlooi, J., Essman, W.B., and Desiderio, D. Macromolecule synthesis in neonatal sheep brain: Effect of prenatal thyroidectomy. *Pediatr. Res.* 1981; 15:507.

Essman, E.J., Ayromlooi, J., Essman, W.B., Tobias, M., and Desiderio, D. Thyrotropin releasing hormone receptors in fetal sheep thyroid. *Pediatr. Res.* 1980; 14:454.

Essman, W.B., Ayromlooi, J., and Essman, E.J. Uptake of biogenic amines by regional synaptosomes from neonatal sheep brain: Effect of *in utero* thyroidectomy. *Physiologist* 1979; 22:69.

Fisher, D.A., Daussault, J.H., Sack, J., and Chopra, I.J. Ontogenesis of hypothalamic-pituitary-thyroid function and metabolism in man, sheep and rat. *Recent Prog. Horm. Res.* 1977; 33:59-116.

Goswami, J., Rao, P.M., and Panda, J.N. Physio-chemical status of hypo-thalamus as affected by hypothyroidism during pregnancy. *Indian J. Exp. Biol.* 1980; 18:5254.

Grilo Reina, A., Jimenez Sanchez, J.R., Mino Fugarolas, G., Moreno Heredia, E., Pera Madrazo, C., Lopez Rubio, F., and Jimenez Pereperez, J.A. Diabetes insipida transitoria tras la extirpacion de carcinoma medular de tiroides. *Medicaina Clin.* (Barcelona) 1980; 75:949-953.

Gripois, D., and Fernandez, C. Influence des hormones thyroidiennes sur l'activite de la monoamine oxydase chez le rat nouveau-ne. *C.R. Acad. Sci.* 1976; 283:1225.

Gripois, D., and Fernandez, C. Thyroxine and propylthiouracil-induced changes in the activity of monamine oxidase in the fetal rat. *Mech. Aging Devel.* 1977; 6:407-412.

Gross, G., Brodde, O.-E., and Schumann, H.J. Effects of thyroid hormone deficiency on pre- and postsynaptic noradrenergic mechanisms in the rat cerebral cortex. *Arch. Int. Pharmacodyn.* 1980; 244:219-230.

Hamburgh, M. An analysis of the action of thyroid hormone on development based on *in vivo* studies. *J. Gen. Comp. Endocrinol.* 1968; 10:198-213.

Harris, R.A., and Loh, H.H. Brain sulfatide and non-lipid sulfate metabolsim in hypothyroid rats. *Res. Comm. Chem. Pathol. Pharmacol.* 1979; 24:169-179.

Hendrich, Ch.E., Porterfield, S.P., and Galton, V.A. Pituitary-thyroid function of fetuses of hypothyroid and growth hormone treated hypothyroid rats. *Horm. Metab. Res.* 1979; 11:362-365.

Hetzel, B.S., and Hay, I.D. Thyroid function, iodine nutrition and fetal brain development. *Clin. Endocrinol.* 1979; 11:445-460.

Hollingsworth, D.R., Belin, R.P., Parker, J.C., Moser, R.J., and McKean, H. Experimental cretinism in lambs: An intrauterine model and thyroid evaluation in surviving lambs. *Johns Hopkins Med. J.* 1975; 137: 116-122.

Holt, A.B., Kerr, G.R., and Cheek, D.B. (1975): Prenatal hypothyroidism and brain composition. *In* D.B. Cheek (Ed.), *Fetal and Postnatal Growth; Hormones and Nutrition.* New York: Wiley, pp. 141-154.

Jacoby, J.H., Mueller, G., and Wurtman, R.J. Thyroid state and brain monoamine metabolism. *Endocrinology* 1975; 97:1332-1335.

Koutras, D.A., Berman, M., Spontouris, J., Rigopoulos, G.A., Koukoulommati, A.S., and Malamos, B. Endemic goiter in Greece: Thyroid hormone kinetics. *J. Clin. Endocrinol. Metab.* 1970; 30:479-487.

Lauder, J.M. Effects of early hypo- and hyperthyroidism on development of rat cerebellar cortex. IV. The parallel fibers. *Brain Res.* 1978; 142: 25-39.

Lauder, J.M. Granule cell migration in developing rat cerebellum. Influence of neonatal hypo- and hyperthyroidism. *Develop. Biol.* 1979; 70: 105-115.

Legrand, J. Influence de l'hypothyroidisme sur la maturation due cortex cérébelleux. *C.R. Acad. Sci.* 1965; 261:544-547.

Mantzos, J.D., Chiotake, L., and Levis, G.M. Biosynthesis and composition of brain glactolipids in normal and hypothyroid rats. *J. Neurochem.* 1973; 21:1207-1213.

McIntosh, G.H., Baghurst, K.I., Potter, B.J., and Hetzel, B.S. Foetal thyroidectomy and brain development in the sheep. *Neuropathol. Appl. Neurobiol.* 1979a; 5:363-376.

McIntosh, G.H., Baghurst, K.I., Potter, B.J., and Hetzel, B.S. Foetal brain development in the sheep. *Neuropathol. Appl. Neurobiol.* 1979b; 5:103-114.

Moonat, L.B.S., Asaad, M.M., and Clarke, D.F. L-thyroxine and monoamine oxidase activity in the kidney and some other organs of the rat. *Res. Commun. Chem. Pathol. Pharmacol.* 1975; 12:765.

Nemeroff, C.B., Lipton, M.A., and Kizer, J.S. Models of neuroendocrine regulation: Use of monosodium glutamate as an investigational tool. *Dev. Neurosci.* 1978; 1:102-109.

Nicholson, J.L., and Altman, J The effects of early hypo- and hyperthy-

roidism on the development of the rat cerebellar cortex. II. Synaptogenesis in the molecular layer. *Brain Res.* 1972; 44:25-36.

Oliver, C., Giraud, P., Gillioz, P., Conte-Devoix, B., and Usategui, R. Brain
TRH levels during development of the rat, in neonatal hypothyroidism
and after caloric deprivation. *Biol. Neonate* 1980; 37:1-7.

Patel, M.S. Influence of neonatal hypothyroidism on the development of
ketone-body-metabolizing enzymes in rat brain. *Biochem. J.* 1979;
184:169-172.

Patel, A.J., Smith, R.M., Kingsbury, A.E., Hunt, A., and Balázs, R. Effects
of the thyroid state on brain development: Muscarinic acetylcholine and
GABA receptors. *Brain Res.* 1980; 198:389-402.

Pesetzky, I. The development of abnormal cerebellar astrocytes in young
hypothyroid rats. *Brain Res.* 1973; 63:456-460.

Querido, A., and Swaab, D.F. (Eds.) (1975): *In Brain Development and
Thyroid Deficiency.* Amsterdam: North Holland Publishing Co.

Rastogi, R.B., and Singhal, R.L. Alterations in brain norepinephrine and
tyrosine hydroxylase activity during experimental hypothyroisidm in
rats. *Brain Res.* 1974; 81:253-266.

Rastogi, R.B., and Singhal, R.L. Influence of neonatal and adult hyperthyroidism on behaviour and biosynthetic capacity for norepinephrine,
dopamine and 5-hydroxytryptamine in rat brain. *J. Pharmacol. Exp.
Ther.* 1976; 198:609-618.

Rastogi, R.B., and Singhal, R.L. The effect of thyroid hormone on serotonergic neurones: Depletion of serotonin in discrete brain areas of
developing hypothyroid rats. *Naunyn-Schmiedeberg's Arch. Pharmacol.*
1978; 304:9-13.

Rastogi, R.B., and Singhal, R.L. Effect of neonatal hypothyroidism and
delayed L-Triiodothyronine treatment on behavioural activity and
norepinephrine and dopamine biosynthetic systems in discrete regions
of rat brain. *Psychopharmacology* 1979; 62:287-293.

Reichlin, S., and Mitnick, M. (1973): Biosynthesis of hypothalamic hypophysiotropic factors. *In* W.L. Ganong and L. Martini (Eds.), *Frontiers
in Neuroendocrinology.* New York: Oxford University Press, pp. 61-88.

Schalock, R.L. Neonatal hypothyroidism: Behavioral, thyroid hormonal and
neuroanatomical effects. *Physiol. Behav.* 1977; 19:489-491.

Shopsin, B., Shenkman, L., Sanghvi, I., and Hollander, C.S. Toward a
relationship between the hypothalamic-pituitary-thyroid axis and the
synthesis of serotonin. *Adv. Biochem. Psychopharm.* 1974; 10:
279-286.

Singhal, R.L., Rastogi, R.B., and Hrdina, P.D. Impaired brain amine
metabolism in neonates during altered states of thyroid function.
Life Sci. 1975; 17:1617-1626.

Smith, R.M., Patel, A.J., Kingsbury, A.E., Hunt, A., and Balazs, R. Effects
of thyroid state on brain development: β-adrenergic receptors and
5'-nucleotidase activity. *Brain Res.* 1980; 198:375-387.

Spinks, A., and Burn, J.H. Thyroid activity and amine oxidase in the liver.
Br. J. Pharmacol. Chemother. 1952; 7:93.

Thorburn, G.P., and Hopkins, P.S. (1972): Thyroid function in the foetal
lamb. *In Foetal and Neonatal Physiology, Proc. Sir Joseph Barcroft
Centenary Symposium.* Cambridge, England: Cambridge University
Press, pp. 488-507.

Verity, M.A., Brown, W.J., Cheung, M., Huntsman, H., and Smith, R. Effects of neonatai ı ypothyroidism on cerebral and cerebellar synaptosome development. *J. Neuroscience Res.* 1976; 2:323-335.

Walravens, P., and Chase, H.P. Influence of thyroid on formation of myelin lipids. *J. Neurochem.* 1969; 16:1477-1484.

5

Thyroid Hormone Actions in the Lung

DIPAK K. DAS
and
HARRY STEINBERG

It is now well established that the lung has many other functions in addition to gas exchange. Lung cells, of which 40 different types have thus far been identified, are capable of performing various metabolic functions (Ballard and Ballard, 1974; Avery, 1968). For example, endothelial cells lining the pulmonary vascular bed have been found to activate angiotensin I to II, inactivate the bradykinin and noradrenalin, inactivate serotonin, and synthesize and degrade prostaglandins (Alabaster and Bakhle, 1972; Ginn and Vane, 1968; Crutchley and Piper, 1974; Steinberg et al., 1975).

The type II alveolar epithelial cell, one of the cells lining the alveolar space, has been found to synthesize dipalmitoyl phosphatidyl choline. This phospholipid comprises a major portion of the pulmonary surface active material necessary to ensure alveolar stability at very low distending pressures (Avery and Mead, 1959; Clements et al., 1961; King and Clements, 1972; Oldenborg and Van Golde, 1977). Phospholipid biosynthesis depends on a number of factors, including lung maturity, availability of substrates, and hormonal factors. For example, glucocorticoids have been shown to stimulate surfactant synthesis, thereby hastening lung maturation (Liggens and Howie, 1972). Additional hormones that affect surfactant synthesis have also been described (Redding et al., 1972; Hamosh and Hamosh, 1972).

The discovery of glucocorticoid receptors in the lung has led to extensive investigations into other receptors and their role in lung growth and development. Most recently, thyroid receptors have been identified in lung and thyroid hormone has been shown to affect surfactant synthesis. The information that will be presented is a summary of what is presently known concerning the role of thyroid hormone in the various aspects of pulmonary growth and development.

THYROID HORMONE IN LUNG

Although thyroid hormones have been postulated to play a role in lung development, little is known about the mechanism of thyroid hormone action on lung metabolism or the actual concentration of this hormone in lung tissue. Recently it was found that the cellular compartment of lung contains an appreciable amount of T_3 (Hitchcock and Reichlin, 1978). Unlike other organs where tissue-to-plasma ratios of T_4 are significant, T_4 was not detected in adult rat lung in this study. Concentration of T_3 in lung was found to be 1.59 ± 0.25 ng/g of lung compared with 2.68 ± 0.25 ng/g in liver and 4.72 ± 0.29 ng/g in kidney (Table 1).

In another study, Obregon and his co-workers (1978) also found appreciable amounts of T_3 in rat lung, and the concentration was greater than that found in the plasma. It appears from these studies that T_3 may be the principal thyroid hormone in the lung. This supports the previous observations that thyroid hormone may have a significant role in the regulation of surfactant synthesis. The stimulatory role of T_3 may act on the *de novo* synthesis of the surface-active lipoprotein in a manner similar to the previously described effects of thyroid hormone in stimulating lipid synthesis (Ingbar et al., 1972).

THYROID HORMONE RECEPTORS

Identification of Receptors in Fetal and Adult Lungs

The biological effects of T_3 and T_4 on target organs are generally believed to be mediated through the binding of these hormones to specific receptors. Nuclear receptors for T_3 have recently been reported in the lungs of adult and fetal animals (Morishige and

Table 1.   Distribution of Thyroxine (T_4) and Triiodothyronine (T_3)
in Adult Rat Lung, Liver, and Kidney*

	Thyroxine		*Triiodothyronine*	
Tissue	*Tissue/Plasma*	*Hormone Concentration (ng/g)*	*Tissue/Plasma*	*Hormone Concentration (ng/g)*
Lung	0.04 ± 0.02	—	2.57 ± 0.40	1.59 ± 0.25
Liver	0.45 ± 0.02	16.89 ± 0.68	4.32 ± 0.40	2.68 ± 0.25
Kidney	0.35 ± 0.03	13.17 ± 0.99	7.62 ± 0.81	4.72 ± 0.29
Plasma	—	38.00 ± 0.49	—	0.62 ± 0.10

*Values represent the average of three or four experiments with their calculated standard errors. Data reproduced from Hitchcock and Reichlin (1978) with permission from *American Review of Respiratory Disease*

Guernsey, 1978; Lindenberg et al., 1978).   Saturable and high-affinity binding of T_3 by nuclei from lung tissue and by cell lines derived from lung have been demonstrated.   In rat lungs saturation analysis under equilibrium conditions demonstrates a single order of high-affinity binding sites with an apparent dissociation constant of 0.254 ± 0.027 nM and an apparent capacity of 249.4 ± 15.5 fmoles/mg DNA.   Incubation of isolated nuclei with ^{125}I-T_3 results in approximately 2400 specific binding sites per cell in fetal rabbit lungs and 1120 sites per cell in adult lung (Table 2).   The affinity of T_3 binding during late fetal life is the same, indicating the presence of thyroid hormone receptors prior to the maturation of alveolar epithelial type II cells.   In L-2 and A-549 cells derived from the type II cells, approximately 2280 and 1580 nuclear sites per cell, respectively, have been reported.

Table 2.   Nuclear Receptor for Thyroid Hormone in Lung and Cell Lines Derived from Lung

	Nuclear Binding of ^{125}I T_3	
Tissues	*Sites/Cell*	*K_D (pM)*
Adult rat lung	900	0.25
Adult rabbit lung	1120	0.54
Fetal rabbit lung	2400	0.50
L-2 cells	2280	0.28
A-549 cells	1580	0.20

Data reproduced from Morishige and Guernsey (1978) and Lindenberg et al. (1978) with permission from Williams & Wilkins

Recent studies have also demonstrated the binding of ^{125}I-T_3 by the nuclei from fetal and neonatal lungs (Das, 1980a). Maximum binding capacity of I-125 T_3 increased with increase in gestational age, but fell significantly after birth (Figure 1). This finding was not observed in neonatal or fetal liver. The binding of T_3 by lung has a specificity similar to that observed in other thyroid hormone-responsive tissues (Oppenheimer et al., 1976). As shown in Table 3, the binding potencies of D-T_3 relative to L-T_3 is 54% whereas the relative affinity for L-T_4 is only 7%. Substitution of an isopropyl group for the 3-iodo group does not affect the binding activity appreciably. In fetal lung little binding activity of L-T_3 was observed for reverse-T_3 (r-T_3), 3,3-diiodothyronine (3,3-L-T_2), and 3,5-dimethyl-3'-isopropyl-L-thyronine (DIMIT). Despite the low binding affinity for DIMIT, the binding activity of this synthetic noniodinated analogue with fetal lung may have practical importance. In contrast to T_3 and T_4, DIMIT can cross the placental barrier and it has been shown that administration of this compound to pregnant rats can prevent fetal goiter (Comite et al., 1978) and induce morphologic and enzymatic changes in fetal liver (Kriz et al., 1978; Benson et al., 1978). Recently it was reported that DIMIT treatment of the pregnant rabbits increases the rate of choline incorporation into lecithin in fetal lung slices (Ballard et al., 1978). Thus maternal administration of this compound may induce thyroid hormone-responsiveness in fetuses through interaction with nuclear binding sites.

Localization of Thyroid Hormone Receptors

Using both direct and indirect immunofluorescence techniques, Wilson and co-workers were able to localize T_3 and T_4 in cultures of cells derived from adult rat type II pulmonary epithelial cells. Two different fluorescent patterns were observed in the cells: (a) nuclear fluorescence accompanied by reticular perinuclear network, and (b) diffuse cytoplasmic accumulations with concentrations around perinuclear cytoplasmic inculsions containing surfactant-associated nonspecific esterases. Using a similar cell line, Lindenberg et al. (1978) demonstrated the presence of specific nuclear T_3 receptors in fetal and adult lungs.

Receptors for thyroid hormone have also been isolated from the mitochondrial fraction of lung. The inner mitochondrial membrane of rat lung was found to contain high-affinity T_3 receptors (K_A =

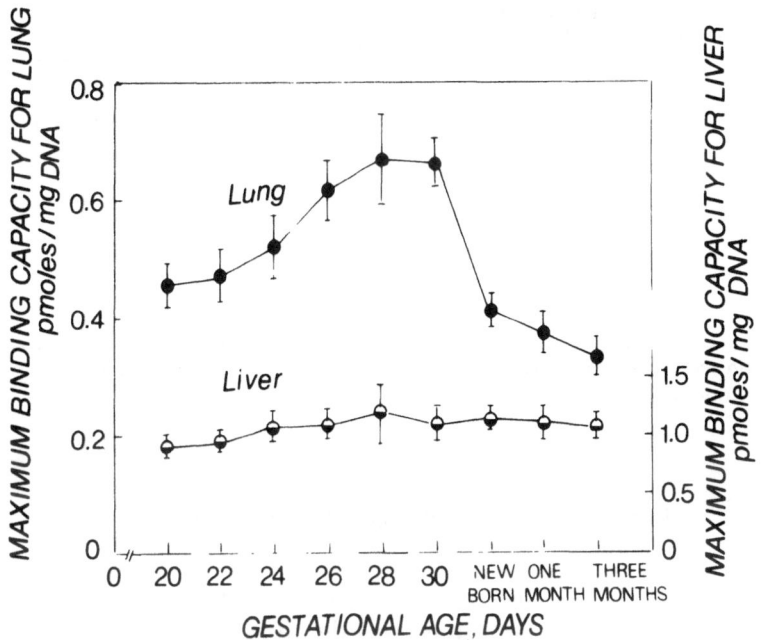

Fig. 1. Comparison of maximum binding capacity of $^{125}I\,T_3$ for lungs (●—●) and livers (○—○) of rabbit fetus. Nuclei from lungs and livers of rabbit fetus were prepared, purified, and incubated with radiolabeled T_3. Binding parameters were assessed by Scatchard analysis of dose-response experiments. Values are MEANS ± SEM. Data reproduced from Das (1980a) with permission from Academic Press.

$1.8 \times 10^{11}\,M^{-1}$) that exhibited low-capacity binding (Sakuruda et al., 1978). This inner matrix of mitochrondria contained approximately 50% lipid, largely phospholipids tentatively identified as lecithin, phosphatidyl ethanolamine, and cardiolipin. Crude mitochondria showed no specific binding for T_3 because of high nonspecific binding. The presence of T_3 receptors in the inner mitochondrial membrane suggests a direct action of thyroid hormone on the mitochondria independent of the nuclear action.

Thus the results from the foregoing experiments suggests that specific binding sites for thyroid hormone, especially T_3, are present in the lung, and that these binding sites are located in the nucleus and specific locations within the mitochondria and cytoplasm. The identification of these receptors in the alveolar type II cell strongly suggests that phospholipid synthesis may be dependent upon the action of thyroid hormone.

Table 3. Relative Affinities of Thyroid Hormone Analogues for Binding
to Nuclei of 28-Day Fetal Rabbit Lung and Adult Rat Lung

Compound	Relative Affinity for Binding	
	Adult Rat	Fetal Rabbit
L-T$_3$	100	100
T$_2$-1 Pr	—	81
D-T$_3$	54	73
L-T$_4$	7	6.7
3,3'-L-T$_2$	0.1	0.19
DIMIT	—	0.15
r-T$_3$	—	0.08

Data reproduced from Morishige and Guernsey (1978) and Lindenberg et al.
(1978) with permission from Williams & Wilkins

Hormonal Control of Receptors in Lung

Recent studies by Guernsey and Morishige (1979) showed that
nuclear T$_3$ binding capacity in lung was depressed significantly in
genetically obese mice, thus suggesting that lung cells are able
genetically to control the number of nuclear T$_3$ receptors in
response to a metabolic state. Studies in our laboratory have shown
that diabetes, hypophysectomy, and thyroidectomy reduce T$_3$
binding capacity of rat lung (Ganguly and Das, 1980). For
example, the apparent binding capacity of the T$_3$ receptors of
lungs of normal animals was found to be 0.321 pmoles/mg DNA
± 0.014 (Table 4). The maximum binding capacity of T$_3$ receptors
for the lungs of diabetic, hypophysectomized, and thyroidectomized rats was 0.224 ± 0.009, 0.195 ± 0.007, and 0.102 ± 0.007
pmoles/mg DNA respectively. However, the binding capacity of
T$_3$ was found to be the same under all these hormonal conditions,
the values for the dissociation constants (K_d) being 256.3 ± 32.4
pM, 269.6 + 38.1 pM, 248.5 ± 40.3 pM, and 260 ± 52.2 pM for
normal, diabetic, hypophysectomized, and thyroidectomized
animals respectively. Although the mechanism by which this
alteration occurs is not clear, it is conceivable that any metabolic
activity occurring in the hormonally deprived states mediated
through T$_3$ and its receptors could be subject to change. The
changes in enzyme activities in pulmonary tissue that have been
observed previously upon T$_3$-mediated stimulation may also be
explained by an altered relationship between T$_3$ and its receptors
(Kumar et al., 1977; Ganguly et al., 1979). Moreover, the loss of
nuclear T$_3$ receptors in certain cases is believed to mediate the

Table 4. Comparison of the L-Triiodothyronine Binding Affinities in Rat Lung Under Different Hormonal Conditions

Hormonal Condition	Maximum Binding Capacity pMoles/mg DNA	Dissociation Constant K_d (pM)
Normal	0.321 ± 0.014	256.3 ± 32.4
Diabetic	0.224 ± 0.009*	269.6 ± 38.1
Hypophysectomized	0.195 ± 0.007*	248.5 ± 40.3
Thyroidectomized	0.102 ± 0.008*	260.0 ± 82.0

*$p < 0.005$

Data presented at 62nd annual meeting of the Endocrine Society, June 1980, Washington, D.C.

expression of hormonal activity (Oppenheimer et al., 1972, 1974). Because of the similarities existing between lung and other thyroid-responsive tissues with respect to the action of thyroid hormones, it can be postulated that the reported regulatory effect of T_3 on lung metabolism may also be mediated by specific T_3 receptors.

MECHANISM OF ACTION

Direct

The mechanisms of action of thyroid hormone in the lung is not understood. Although the lung has many functions other than gas exchange, the actions of thyroid hormone have been investigated principally in surfactant metabolism. Gross and his co-workers (1979) reported stimulation of the incorporation of choline into phosphatidylcholine after exposing lung explants of fetal rats to thyroxine. When the distribution of radioactivity from ^{3}H-acetate in the phospholipid fractions was studied in the explants, marked differences were observed in the pattern distribution of radio-activity between thyroxine-treated explants and dexamethasone-treated explants. Corticosteroids stimulated surfactant phospho-lipids by increasing phosphatidylcholine and phosphatidylglycerol synthesis, presumably by activating in part the enzymes of deacylation/reacylation pathway (Das et al., 1982). On the other hand, thyroxine stimulated phosphatidylcholine synthesis but inhibited phosphatidylglycerol synthesis. Smith and Torday (1974) also reported increased incorporation of choline into phosphatidyl-choline after exposure of cultures of mixed cells from the lungs of fetal rabbits to thyroxine, but they were unable to demonstrate any stimulation of the methylation pathway. However, Adamson and Bowden (1975) and Funkhouser and Hughes (1977) could not stimulate the incorporation of palmitate into lung tissue in explants from fetal rats by either thyroxine or triiodothyronine.

Although controversy exists regarding the mechanism of action of thyroid hormone on phospholipid synthesis, it is clear that the alveolar epithelial type II cell, the putative cell of origin of the surfactant, seems to be the principal target for this hormone. The major substrate for phospholipid synthesis is glucose, which may be utilized in a number of ways (Figure 2). Lungs may use glucose either from circulating glucose or from the breakdown of glycogen. Evidence suggests that the latter may be a substrate for phospholipid synthesis. For example, glycogen content in fetal lung decreases at the same time that the rate of phosphatidylcholine synthesis increases (Kikkawa, 1971; Maniscalco, 1978). Moreover, corticosteroids associated with lung development decrease glycogen content in lung also. Acetyl CoA and glycerophosphate derived from glucose or glycogen ultimately lead to the formation of phosphatidic acid. This subsequently yields diglyceride, which serves then as a source for the glycerol moiety of dipalmitoylphosphatidylglycerol (Figure 2).

The biologic effects of T_3 and T_4 in thyroid hormone-responsive tissue are mediated to the binding of these hormones to specific receptors. Figure 3 represents a schematic of this process as proposed by Ballard (Ballard, 1978). In the nucleus the hormone binds tightly to receptor proteins residing on chromatin thereby initiating new RNA synthesis, which then enhances protein synthesis and subsequently exerts a physiologic effect. A close correlation exists between the occupancy of nuclear sites by T_3 with the activity of inducible enzymes in thyroid hormone target tissues (Oppenheimer et al., 1976). Acetyl CoA is the source for *de novo* synthesis of fatty acids. Two enzymes involved in fatty acid synthesis in the lung, acetyl CoA carboxylase and fatty acid synthetase, are activated by T_3 (Kumar et al., 1977; Das, 1980a,b). A correlation has been demonstrated between the relative rates of fatty acid synthesis and the maximum binding capacity of T_3 in fetal lungs (Figure 4). The pulmonary nuclear uptake of ^{125}I-T_3 increases with gestational age, as does the synthesis of pulmonary fatty acids. The presence of nuclear receptors for thyroid hormone in mammalian lung has been described, and therefore the properties of T_3 binding by lung closely resemble those described for other thyroid responsive tissue (Morishige and Guernsey, 1978; Oppenheimer et al., 1976).

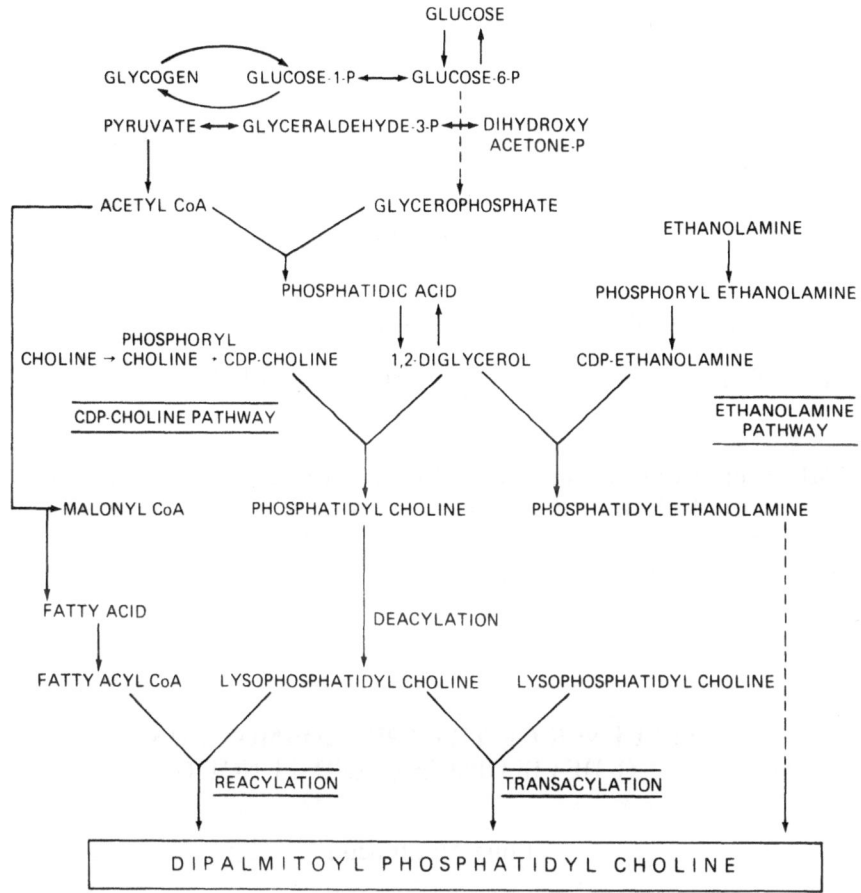

Fig. 2. Pathways for the biosynthesis of lung surfactant.

Indirect

Stimulation of the β-adrenergic system has been shown to potentiate surfactant release into the alveolar space. For example, isoxsuprine has been used to achieve lung stability by enhancing surface activity, presumably by increasing the lecithin to sphingo-myelin ratio (Corbet et al., 1977; Enhorning et al., 1977). Although there is no evidence that thyroid hormone stimulates adrenergic sites in the lung, there are data to support this concept in other tissues (Ciarldi and Marinetti, 1977; Williams et al., 1977). Thyroid-responsive β-adrenergic receptor sites have been described in neonatal rat heart cells where a corresponding increase in cyclic

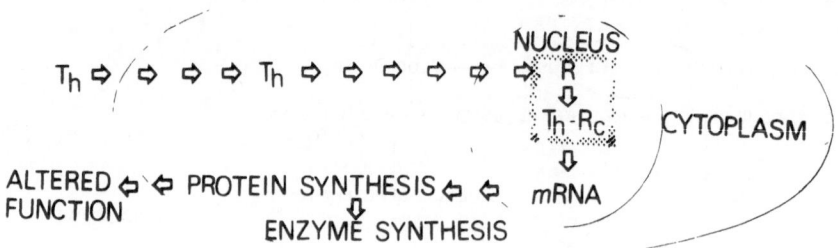

PROPOSED MODEL FOR THYROID HORMONE ACTION IN LUNG

Fig. 3. Proposed model for the biosynthesis of lung surfactant.

AMP to epinephrine was noted (Tsai and Chen, 1978). Thus, in spite of the lack of evidence at this time supporting an indirect mode of action of thyroid hormone in the lung, it does seem plausible from the studies in other organ systems that this hormone could alter cellular function in the lung by interacting with the adrenergic system.

INFLUENCE OF THYROID HORMONE ON LUNG DEVELOPMENT AND FUNCTION

Lung Maturation

It is well known that thyroid hormone has a profound effect on fetal growth and development. This effect on the central nervous system and musculoskeletal system has been well described (Schapiro, 1966, Schapiro, 1968; Best and Ducon, 1969; Simillia and Anitolainen, 1970). Only recently has the role of this hormone been investigated in fetal lung development (Wigglesworth, 1979; Stern, 1979). Wu et al. (1973) were the first to use thyroxine to stimulate maturation of fetal rabbit lung. Thyroxine was administered either to the mother or directly to the fetus within the amniotic sack. The lungs of the fetuses injected directly had a higher surface activity than controls as evidenced by a higher bubble stability ratio and increased air retention in the lungs after inflation. This increase in lung stability was shown to be associated with accelerated maturation of the lung, specifically of the type II alveolar epithelial cells. These type II cells contained increased

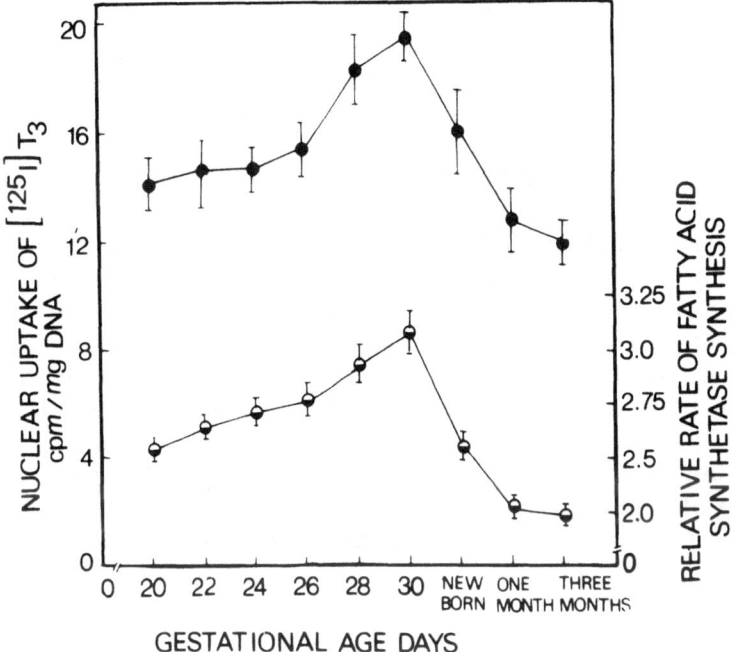

Fig. 4. Comparison of nuclear uptake of ^{125}I T$_3$ (●—●) and relative rate of fatty acid synthetase synthesis (●—○) by fetal rabbit lung [for details of the methods see Das (1980a)]. Data reproduced from Das, 1980a, with permission from Academic Press.

number of lamella bodies, which are presumably the source of lung surfactant (Klaus et al., 1962; Kikkawa et al., 1965; Morgan, 1971). The administration of thyroxine to the mother resulted in little change in lung development because thyroxine generally does not cross the placenta (Grumbach and Werner, 1956).

Sack and his colleagues (1979) have demonstrated that thyroxine administered intraamniotically to humans results in absorption of this hormone by the premature human fetus. Twenty-four hours following the intraamniotic administration of 250 μg of T$_4$, the mean cord serum concentration in 13 premature newborns was found to be 17 ± 2.1 μg/100 ml as compared with a control value of 11.6 ± 0.9. However, this hyperthyroxineemia was only transient.

The effect of intraamniotic thyroxine injection on fetal lung development was reported by Mashiach et al. (1978). These investigators injected 200 μg of thyroxine directly into the amniotic sack in eight women of high-risk pregnancies where premature delivery was indicated. Fetal lung maturity was evalu-

ated by using a microviscosity parameter in the amniotic fluid
(Shinizky et al., 1976). The microviscosity values dropped
significantly as a result of the thyroxine administration, indicating
fetal lung maturity. In an additional study using the technique
of fluorescence polarization (Shinizky et al., 1976) the same
investigators reported significant improvement in the degree of
lung maturity after the intraamniotic injection of thyroxine
(Mashiach et al., 1979). Perhaps of greater significance was the
fact that none of the premature newborns developed evidence of
respiratory distress syndrome. The changes in the intraamniotic
fluid as a result of thyroid hormone administration may have been
the result of the previously described effect of an increased number
of lamellar bodies in the type II epithelial cell and the increased
amount of phosphatidylcholine in lung lavage (Redding et al.,
1972; Rooney and Motoyama, 1977). Interestingly, a low concentration of triiodothyronine and thyroxine in core blood is
generally present in newborn infants suffering from respiratory
distress syndrome (Cuestas et al., 1976).

Cholinergic System

Cholinergic development in the embryonic lung occurs as a
result of the migration of neuroblasts from the vagus to the carina
of the trachea. The formation of neuroepithelial cells by the
maturing ganglia promotes growth of nerve fibers to the tracheal
epithelium. In an *in vitro* study using embryonic lung dissociated
from the central nervous system, Morikawa et al. (1978) observed
accelerated nerve fiber growth and differentiation of ganglia as a
result of thyroxine treatment. Cross sections of the tracheal ring
from the level of the carina were cultured at $37°C$ for one to two
days. After the culture was incubated with thyroxine, the tissue
was stained for acetylcholine esterase (Karnovsky and Roots,
1964). Ganglia were seen to mature in nerves extended from the
ganglia to the epithelium. Submucosalaganglia were also observed
(Figure 5). In controls where no thyroxine was added, no such
accelerated development was observed.

Collagen Synthesis

There are little data dealing with hormonal effects on the
interstitial compartment of the lung. The little that is known

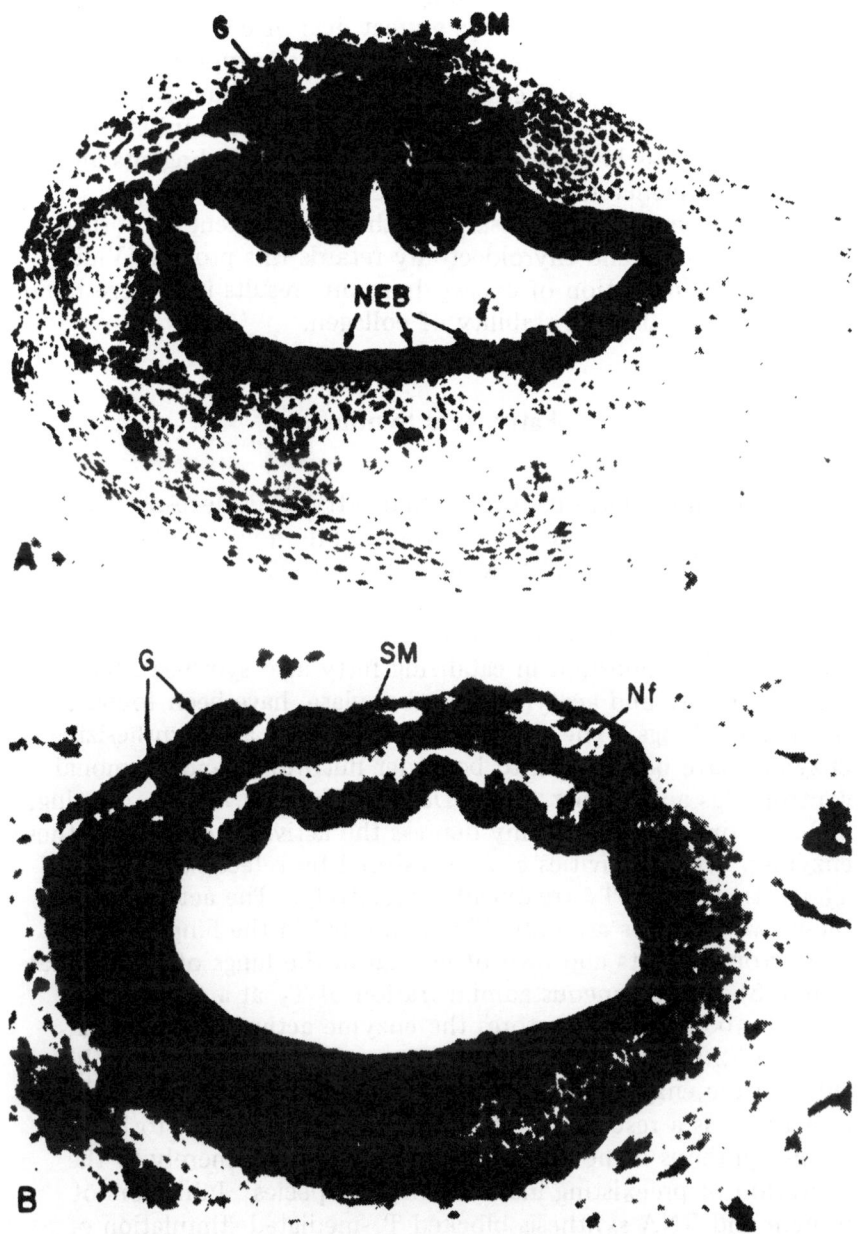

Fig. 5. Seventeen-day tracheal ring *in vitro* exposed to 1 g/ml thyroxine for 24 hours. Ganglia (G) differentiate and nerve fibers (Nf) appear (B). Nervous development is accelerated in comparison with that observed in control tracheal rings (A). Data reproduced from Morikawa et al. (1978) with permission from Grune & Stratton.

suggests that thyroid hormone may have an effect on one of the components. The lung contains a great deal of collagen. The cartilage in the bronchi contains type II, vessels type I and III, and most of the supportive connective tissue collagen is probably type I (Crystal, 1974). Variation of total collagen content in the lung with age has been reported and several external agents are known to influence these age-related changes. For example, thyroxine seems to be necessary for the development of normal temperal changes and thyroidectomy retards this process (Vidik, 1979). Administration of excess thyroxine results in a more rapid increase of the thermal stability of collagen.

Fatty Acid Synthesis

Recent studies have confirmed that fatty acids necessary for pulmonary surfactant may be synthesized *de novo* by the lung (Schiller and Bensch, 1971; Kumar et al., 1977; Das, 1978). For example, a high-speed supernatant fraction of rat lung homogenate is able to synthesize fatty acids by the malonyl CoA pathway. Two enzymes important in catalizing fatty acid synthesis, fatty acid synthetase and acetyl CoA carboxylase, have been found in mammalian lungs. The activities of these fatty acid synthesizing enzymes have been found to be under nutritional and hormonal control (Das and Kumar, 1975; Das and Ganguly, 1978). Fasting, diabetes, or hypophysectomy depress the activities of both of these enzymes. Their activities can be restored by refeeding, insulin or T_3 treatment, and T_3 treatment respectively. The activities of these two enzymes are only 66% of normal in the lungs of hypophysectomized rats and 33% of normal in the lungs of diabetic rats (Table 5). Subcutaneous administration of T_3 at a dose of 100 μg/100 g body weight restores the enzyme activities to normal levels in 72 hours. Repeated injections with T_3 at 0 and 72 hours enhance the enzyme activities to supranormal levels. Enhancement of activity as a result of T_3 treatment has been shown to be due to the synthesis of new enzyme proteins and not merely to the activation of preexisting inactive enzyme species. Inhibitors of protein and RNA synthesis blocked T_3-mediated stimulation of fatty acid synthetase and acetyl CoA carboxylase. In addition, T_3-mediated stimulation of the relative rates of synthesis of fatty acid synthetase follow the same pattern as the specific activities of this enzyme in lung (Table 6). The specific activities of fatty acid synthetase in the lungs of the diabetic and hypophysectomized

Table 5. Response of Lung Fatty Acid Synthesizing System
of Normal, Diabetic, and Hypophysectomized Rats to T_3

Hormonal Condition	Acetyl CoA Carboxylase (nmoles Malonyl CoA Formed/ Minute)	Fatty Acid Synthetase (nmoles NADPH Oxidized/ Minute)
Normal	15.0 ± 0.9	131.0 ± 3.0
Normal + T_3	18.4 ± 1.7	162.0 ± 15.0
Normal + T_3, repeated	19.0 ± 1.0	163.0 ± 6.0
Diabetic	5.4 ± 0.2	46.6 ± 1.5
Diabetic + T_3	14.8 ± 0.8	122.0 ± 17.0
Diabetic + T_3, repeated	17.2 ± 1.8	141.0 ± 23.0
Hypophysectomized	10.5 ± 0.9	93.6 ± 8.0
Hypophysectomized + T_3	14.5 ± 2.4	118.6 ± 19.5
Hypophysectomized + T_3, repeated	18.0 ± 3.6	137.0 ± 21.0

Results are MEANS $\pm$ SEM of at least two sets, each set containing two animals.
Part of the data reproduced from Kumar et al. (1977) with permission from
Academic Press

rats increased to the same extent after T_3 treatment as a stimulation
of the relative rate of enzyme synthesis. Although T_3 enhances
the rate of synthesis of these two enzymes involved in surfactant
synthesis, the mechanism of induction is not understood.

Prostaglandin Synthesis

Prostaglandins consist of a group of oxygenated fatty acid
derivatives with hormone-like activity. In mammalian lung it has
been suggested that they may play a role in the contractuity of
blood vessels and airways, and it has been shown that they may
participate in the control of collagen production (Mathe et al.,
1977a, 1977b; Hyman et al., 1978; DuComb et al., 1978; Wahl
et al., 1977). Prostaglandins have also been shown to affect the
growth of lung fibroblasts (Taylor and Polgar, 1977). Adult lungs
are capable of synthesizing as well as degrading a number of
prostaglandins (Smith et al., 1973; Farrell, 1977). Recently,
Taylor et al. (1979) studied the effect of thyroid hormone on
prostaglandin production by fetal and adult type II alveolar
epithelial cells. The production of prostaglandin E as well as of
$F_{2\alpha}$ was inhibited considerably by thyroxine. Production of
prostaglandin E and $F_{2\alpha}$ was 9 ± 0.5 and 10 ± 0.4 ng/ml in control
lung organotypic cultures. In thyroxine-treated cultures the pro-

Table 6. Effect of T_3 on the Relative Rates of Synthesis of Lung Fatty Acid
Synthetase in Diabetic and Hypophysectomized Rats

Hormonal Status	Specific Activity nmoles NADPH Oxidized per Minute per Milligram Protein	(A) Total Soluble Protein (CPM/Lung) $\times 10^{-5}$	(B) Total Fatty Acid Synthetase (CPM/Lung) $\times 10^{-3}$	$\frac{B}{A} \times 10^2$ Relative Rate
Diabetic	5.6	1.58	2.02	1.28
Diabetic + T_3	15.0	2.77	9.64	3.48
Hypophysectomized	6.2	1.63	2.21	1.35
Hypophysectomized + T_3	14.7	2.85	8.86	3.11

Two rats were used in each group. Each rat was given 50 μCi L-^{3}H leucine/100 g
body weight and sacrificed after 2 hours; 105,000 g supernatant were prepared
and counts/minute/milligram protein were determined as described
previously (Das, 1980a)

duction of these two types of prostaglandins were only 1.8 ± 0.3
and 1.0 ± 0.5 ng/ml. Similar observations were noted by Moore
and Hoult (1978), who reported that prostaglandin $F_{2\alpha}$ and E_2
degradation was depressed by 40.3 and 41.8%, respectively, in
hyperthyroid rats. The authors concluded that thyroxine treatment decreases the intracellular levels of 15-prostaglandin
dehydrogenase either by reducing the rate of enzyme synthesis or
by accelerating its degradation.

Thus it seems that thyroid hormone may affect prostaglandin
concentration in mammalian lungs and evidence has been presented
that suggests that this hormone can affect both synthesis and
degradation. The mechanism of action of thyroid hormone in
this instance is again not well understood, and it seems possible
that it is interacting either directly with a prostaglandin receptor
or indirectly by affecting fatty acid synthesis or by stimulating
the adrenergic system.

Permeability of the Lung to Drugs

The lung can absorb drugs from both the alveolar surface and
the capillary bed. A review of the subject is beyond the scope of
this brief discussion and the reader is referred to presentations by
Schanker and his colleagues. The effect of thyroid hormone on the

permeability of the lung to drugs had been investigated, but not to any great extent. Lipid-insoluble compounds such as p-aminohippuric acid, tetraethylammonium, and mannitol are absorbed more rapidly by younger rats under the age of 12 days than by 18-day or older rats (Hemberger and Schanker, 1978). This would suggest a change in the lung's permeability characteristics with increasing age. In terms of a lipid-pore model of some membrane (Schanker, 1978) lipid-insoluble compounds can penetrate the membrane principally by diffusing through small aqueous pores, which suggests that an age-related change in permeability reflects an alteration in the porosity of the absorbing membrane. In their study, Hemberger and Schanker injected 1 or 2 μg/g of thyroxine intraperitoneally into rats during the first four days of life and measured the pulmonary absorption of drugs in those animals at ages 6, 12, and 18 days. In the thyroxine-treated rats the absorption rate for lipid-insoluble compounds declined between the ages of 6 and 12 days, whereas the decline occurred between 12 and 18 days of age in controls. Thus these results suggest that thyroxine produces an alteration in normal age related patterns of pulmonary absorption, which probably reflects acceleration in the maturation of the neonatal lung.

THYROID HORMONE, PULMONARY MECHANICS, AND GAS EXCHANGE

Severe hypothyroidism (myxedema) has been reported to result in impaired lung mechanics and hypoventilation. Wilson and Bedell (1960) found a reduced vital capacity (the amount of air an individual can expel from the lungs after a complete expiration) in obese hypothyroid patients, and attributed this finding to an impairment in respiratory muscle. The pulmonary diffusing capacity was also found to be markedly impaired and evidence that this was due directly to the metabolic state was the improvement in this parameter after treatment. The cause of this abnormality is not known but may have been related to an ventilation-perfusion imbalance, diminished cardiac output, or increased capillary permeability.

Hyperthyroidism also results in a reduced vital capacity, probably attributable to muscle weakness and a reduced diffusing capacity (Stein et al., 1961; Massey et al., 1967). Pulmonary compliance, a measure of the lung elasticity, seems also to be reduced. Although it was thought that muscle weakness accounted for the reduction in lung volumes, Freedman (1978) has observed improved lung function in patients treated for thyrotoxicosis without concomitant changes in pulmonary performance.

CONCLUSIONS

The evidence that thyroid hormone plays a role in lung growth and development seems clear. Much of this evidence, however, is based on subcellular preparations, isolated cell systems, and animal experiments. More of the experiments, such as the ones dealing with surfactant maturation, will be necessary before clinical application is warranted. The systemic effects of thyroid hormone on the entire organism are diverse and specific interpretations as to mechanisms will be difficult.

ACKNOWLEDGMENT

The authors would like to thank Dr. Manik Ganguly of New York University Medical Center for his invaluable aid in some of the studies and Mrs. Lois Hirsch for her secretarial assistance.

REFERENCES

Adamson, Y.R., and Bowden, D.H. Reaction of cultured and fetal lung to prednisolone and thyroxine. *Arch. Pathol.* 1975; 99:80–85.
Alabaster, V. A., and Bakhle, Y.S. The inactivation of bradykinin in the pulmonary circulation of isolated lungs. *Br. J. Pharmacol.* 1972; 45: 299–309.
Avery, M.E. (Ed.) (1968): *The Lung and Its Disorders in the Newborn Infant.* Philadelphia: W.B. Saunders Co. 1st edition.
Avery, M.E., and Mead, J. Surface properties in relation to atelectasis and hyaline membrane disease. *Am. J. Dis. Child.* 1959; 97:517–521.
Bakhle, Y.S., and Vane, J.R. Pharmacokinetic function of the pulmonary circulation. *Physiol. Rev.* 1974; 54:1007–1045.
Ballard, P.L., and Ballard, R.A. Cytoplasmic receptor for flucocorticoids in lung of the human fetus and neonate. *J. Clin. Invest.* 1974; 53: 477–486.
Ballard, P.L., Brehier, A., Benson, B.J., Kriz, B.M., and Jorgenson, E.C. Transplacental effects of a thyroxine analog on phospholipid synthesis in fetal rabbit lung. *Pediat. Res.* 1978; 12:558.
Ballard, P.L. (1978) Hormonal regulation of surfactant in fetal life. *In*

Mead Johnson Symposium on Perinatal and Developmental Medicine. no. 14, pp. 25-39.

Barker, S.B., and Lewis, W.J. Thyroxine analog effects on succinate and malate oxidation in vitro. *Fed. Proc.* 1958; 15:8-9.

Beahrs, O.H., and Sakulsky, S.B. Surgical thyroidectomy in the management of exophthalmic goiter. *Arch. Surg.* 1968; 96:512-515.

Beatson, G.T. On the treatment of inoperable cases of carcinoma of the mamma. Suggestions for a new method of treatment with illustrative guesses. *Lancet* 1896; 2:104-107.

Benson, M.C., Liu, J.P., Huang, Y.P., Burger, A., and Rilvin, R.S. Differential effects of triiodothyronine and 3.5-dimethyl-3'-isopropyl-L-thyronine treatment of maternal rats upon hepatic L-triiodothyronine aminotransferase activity in fetal rats. *Endocrinology* 1978; 102:562-567.

Best, M.M., and Ducon, C.H. Accelerated maturation and persistent growth impairment in the rat resulting from thyroxine administration in the neonatal period. *J. Lab. Clin. Med.* 1969; 73:135-143.

Brown, E.A.B. The localization, metabolism and effects of drugs and toxicants in lung. *Drug Metab. Rev.* 1974; 3:33-87.

Ciarldi, T., and Marinetti, G.V. Thyroxine and propyl-thiouracil effects in vivo on alpha and beta adrenergic receptors in rat heart. *Biochem. Biophys. Res. Commun.* 1977; 74:984-991.

Clements, J.A., Hustead, R.F., Johnson, R.P., and Gribetz, I. Pulmonary surface tension and alveolar stability. *J. Appl. Physiol.* 1961; 16:444-450.

Comite, F., Burrow, G.N., and Jorgensen, E.C. Thyroid hormone analogs and fetal goiter. *Endocrinology* 1978; 102:1670-1674.

Corbet, A.J.S., Flax, P., and Rudolph, A.J. Role of autonomic nervous system controlling surface tension in fetal rabbit lungs. *J. Appl. Physiol.* 1977; 43:1039-1045.

Crutchley, D.J., and Piper, P.J. Prostaglandin inactivation in guinea pig lung and its inhibition. *Br. J. Pharmacol.* 1974; 52:197-203.

Crystal, R.G. Lung collagen: Definition, diversity and development. *Fed. Proc.* 1974; 33:2248-2255.

Cuestas, R.A., Lindall, A., and Engel, R.R. Low thyroid hormones and respiratory distress syndrome of the newborn. *N. Engl. J. Med.* 1976; 295:297-302.

Das, D.K. Regulation of hepatic fatty acid synthesizing enzymes of diabetic animals by thyroid hormones. *Arch. Biochem. Biophys.* 1980a; 203:25-36.

Das, D.K. Fatty acid synthesis in fetal lung. *Biochem. Biophys. Res. Commun.* 1980b; 92:867-875.

Das, D.K. Effect of feeding glucose and fructose on the pulmonary fatty acid biosynthesis of diabetic animals. *Am. Rev. Resp. Dis.* 1978; 117:326.

Das, D.K., and Kumar, S. Nutritional and hormonal variations alter de novo fatty acid synthesis in mammalian lung. *Fed. Proc.* 1975; 34:2577.

Das, D.K., and Ganguly, M. Diabetes, hypophysectomy and thyroidectomy reduces L-triiodothyronine binding capacity of rat lung. *Endocrinology* 1981; 109:296-300.

Das, D.K., and Ganguly, M. Hormonal regulation of pulmonary fatty acid synthesis. *Am. Rev. Resp. Dis.* 1978; 117:326.

Das, D.K., Ayromlooi, J., Desiderio, D., Tobias, M., and Steinberg, H. Effect of dexamethasone on the synthesis of dipalmitoyl phosphatidylcholine. *Dev. Pharmacol. Therap.* 1982; 3:55-64.

Douglas, W.H.J., Redding, R.A., and Stein, M. The lamellar substructure of osmiophilic inclusion bodies present in rat type II alveolar pneumonocytes. *Tissue and Cell* 1975; 7:137-142.

DuComb, M., Polgar, P., and Franzblau, C. The effect of prostaglandins on the production of collagen in human embryo lung fibroblast in culture. *Prostaglandin* 1978; 15:708-712.

Dunn, J.T., and Chapman, E.M. Rising incidence of hypothyroidism after radioactive iodine therapy in thyrotoxicosis. *N. Engl. J. Med.* 1964; 271:1037-1042.

Enhorning, G., Chamberlain, D., Contreras, C., Burgoyne, R., and Robertson, B. Isoxsuprine induced release of pulmonary surfactant in the rabbit fetus. *Am. J. Obstet. Gynec.* 1977; 129:197-202.

Farrell, P.M. Fetal lung development and the influence of glucocorticoids on pulmonary surfactant. *J. Steroid. Biochem.* 1977; 8:463-470.

Freedman, S. Lung volumes and distensibility and maximum respiratory pressures in thyroid disease before and after treatment with carbimazole or L-thyroxine when the patients were clinically and biochemically euthyroid. *Thorax* 1978; 33(6):785-790.

Funkhouse, J.D., and Hughes, E.R. Glucocorticoids and fetal lung development. *J. Steroid Biochem.* 1977; 8:519-524.

Ganguly, M., Das, D.K., and Basak, K. Regulation of pulmonary surfactant synthesis by triiodothyronine and dexamethasone. *Fed. Proc.* 1979; 38:235.

Ganguly, M., and Das, D.K. (1980): Hormonal regulation of pulmonary L-triiodothyronine binding capacity. Presented at 62nd Annual Meeting of the Endocrine Society, June 1980, Washington, D.C., abstract #597.

Ginn, R., and Vane, J.R. Disappearance of catecholamines from the pulmonary circulation. *Nature* (London) 1968; 219:740-742.

Gluck, G.E., and McLean, A.A. A preliminary investigation of the hormonal control of the hexose monophosphate oxidative pathway. *Biochem. J.* 1955; 61:390-397.

Gluck, L., Scribney, M., and Kulovich, M.V. The biochemical development of surface activity in mammalian lung. II. The biosynthesis of phospholipids in the lung of the developing rabbit fetus and newborn. *Pediat. Res.* 1967; 1:247-265.

Gross, I., Wilson, C.M., and Ingelson, L.D. Comparison of the effects of dexamethasone and thyroxine on phospholipid synthesis by fetal rat lung in organ culture. *Pediat. Res.* 1979; 13:535.

Grumbach, M.M., and Werner, S.C. Transfer of thyroid hormone across human placenta at term. *J. Clin. Endocrinol.* 1956; 16:1392-1395.

Guernsey, D.L., and Morishige, W.K. Na^+ pump activity and nuclear T_3 receptors in tissues of genetically obese (ob/ob) mice. *Metabolism* 1979; 28:629-632.

Hamosh, M., and Hamosh, P. The effect of prolactin on the lecithin content of fetal rabbit lung. *J. Clin. Invest.* 1977; 59:1002-1005.

Hemberger, J.A., and Schanker, L.S. Pulmonary absorption of drugs in the neonatal rat. *Am. J. Physiol.* 1978; 234:C191-C197.

Hitchcock, K.R., and Reichlin, S. Thyroid hormones in the adult rat lung. *Am. Rev. Res. Dis.* 1978; 117:807-810.

Hoch, F.L. Biochemical actions of thyroid hormones. *Physiol. Rev.* 1962; 42:605-673.

Hyman, A.L., Spannhake, E.W., and Kadowitz, P.J. Prostaglandins and the lung. *Am. Rev. Resp. Dis.* 1978; 117:111-136.

Ingbar, S.H., and Woebar, K.A. (1972): The thyroid gland. *In* R.H. Williams (Ed.), *Textbook of Endocrinology*, 5th ed. Philadelphia: W.B. Saunders Co., p. 95.

Kaliner, M., Orange, R.P., and Austen, K.F. Immunological release of histamine and slow-reacting substance and anaphylaxis from human lung. IV. Enhancement of cholinergic and α-adrenergic stimulation. *J. Exp. Med.* 1972; 136:556-567.

Kapdi, C.C., and Wolfe, J.N. Breast cancer: Relationship to thyroid supplements for hypothyroidism. *JAMA* 1976; 236:1124-1127.

Karnovsky, M.J., and Roots, L. A direct coloring thiocholine method for cholinesterase. *J. Histochem. Cytochem.* 1964; 12:219-221.

Kikkawa, Y., Kaibara, M., Motoyama, E.K., Onzalesi, M.M., and Cook, C.D. Morphologic development of fetal rabbit lung and its acceleration with cortisol. *Am. J. Pathol.* 1971; 64:423-433.

Kikkawa, Y., Motoyama, E.K., and Cook, C.D. The ultrastructure of the lung of lambs. The relationship of osmiophilic inclusions and alveolar lining layer to fetal maturation and experimentally produced respiratory distress. *Am. J. Pathol.* 1965; 47:877-903.

King, R.J., and Clements, J.A. Surface active materials from dog lung. II. Composition and physiological correlations. *Am. J. Physiol.* 1972; 223:715-726.

Klaus, M., Rein, O.K., Tooley, W.H., Piel, C., and Clements, J.A. Alveolar epithelial cell mitochondria as a source of the surface active lung lining. *Science* 1962; 137:750-751.

Kriz, B.M., Jones, A.L., and Jorgensen, E.C. Effects of a thyroid hormone analog on fetal rat hepatocyte ultrastructure and microsomal function. *Endocrinology* 1978; 102:712-722.

Kumar, S., Das, D.K., Dorfman, A.E., and Asato, N. Stimulation of the synthesis of hepatic fatty acid synthesizing enzymes of hypophysectomized rats by 3,5,3'-L-triiodothyronine. *Arch. Biochem. Biophys.* 1977; 178:507-516.

Liggins, G.C., and Howie, R.N. A controlled trial of antepartum glucocorticoid treatment for prevention of the respiratory distress syndrome in premature infants. *Pediatrics* 1972; 50:515-525.

Lindenberg, J.A., Brehier, A., and Ballard, P.L. Triiodothyronine nuclear binding in fetal and adult rabbit lung and cultured lung cells. *Endocrinology* 1978; 103:1725-1731.

Longenecker, G.L., and Huggins, C.G. (1977): Biochemistry of the pulmonary angiotensin-converting enzyme. *In* Y.S. Bakhle and J.R. Vane (Eds.), *Metabolic Function of the Lung.* New York: Marcel Dekker, Inc., pp. 55-83.

Maniscalco, W.M., Wilson, C.M., Gross, I., et al. Development of glycogen and phospholipid metabolism in fetal and newborn rat lung. *Biochim. Biophys. Acta.* 1978; 530:333-346.

Maniscalco, W.M., Wilson, C.M., and Gross, I. Influence of aminophylline and cyclic AMP on glycogen metabolism in fetal rat lung in organ culture. *Pediat. Res.* 1979; 13:1319-1322.

Mashiach, S., Barkai, G., Sack, J., et al. Enhancement of fetal lung maturity by intraamniotic administration of thyroid hormone. *Am. J. Obstet. Gynec.* 1978; 13:289.

Mashiach, S., Barkai, G., Sack, J., et al. The effect of intra-amniotic thyroxine administration on fetal lung maturity in man. *J. Perinat. Med.* 1979; 7:161-170.

Massey, D.G., Becklake, M.R., McKenzie, J.M., and Bates, D.V. Circulatory and ventilatory response to exercise in thyrotoxicosis. *N. Engl. J. Med.* 1967; 276:1104-1112.

Mathe, A.A., Hedqvist, P., Strandberg, K., and Leslie, C.A. Aspects of prostaglandin function in the lung (first of two parts). *N. Engl. J. Med.* 1977a; 296:850-855.

Mathe, A.A., Hedqvist, P., Strandberg, K., and Leslie, C.A. Aspects of prostaglandin function in the lung. *N. Engl. J. Med.* 1977b; 296: 910-914.

Moore, P.K., and Hoult, J.R.S. Experimental hyperthyroidism in rats suppresses in vitro prostaglandin metabolism in lung and kidney. *Prostaglandins* 1978; 16:335-349.

Moossa, A.R., Price Evans, D.A., and Brewer, A.C. Thyroid status and breast cancer. Reappraisal of an old relationship. *Ann. Roy. Coll. Surg. Engl.* 1973; 52:178-191.

Morgan, T.E. Pulmonary surfactant. *N. Engl. J. Med.* 1971; 284:1185-1192.

Morikawa, Y., Donahoe, P.K., and Hendren, W.H. Cholinergic nerve development of fetal lung in vitro. *J. Ped. Surg.* 1978; 13:653-661.

Morishige, W.K., and Guernsey, D.L. Triiodothyronine receptors in rat lung. *Endocrinology* 1978; 102:1628-1632.

Munoz, J.M., Gorman, C.A., Elveback, L.R., and Wentz, J.R. Incidence of malignant neoplasms of all types in patients with Graves' disease. *Arch. Intern. Med.* 1978; 138:944-947.

Obregon, J., DeEscobar, G.M., and Del Rey, F.E. Concentrations of triiodo-L-thyronine in the plasma and tissues of normal rats determined by radioimmunoassay: Comparison with results obtained by an isotopic equillibrium technique. *Endocrinology* 1978; 103:2145-2153.

Odlenborg, V., and Van Golde, L.M.G. The enzymes of phosphatidylcholine biosynthesis in the fetal mouse lung. Effects of dexamethasone. *Biochim. Biophys. Acta* 1977; 489:454-465.

Oppenheimer, J.H., Schwartz, H.L., Surks, M.I., et al. Nuclear receptors and the initiation of thyroid hormone action. *Rec. Prog. Horm. Res.* 1976; 32:529-535.

Oppenheimer, J.H., Koerner, D., Schwartz, H.L., and Surks, M.I. Specific nuclear triiodothyronine binding sites in rat liver and kidney. *J. Clin. Endocrinol. Metab.* 1972; 35:330-334.

Oppenheimer, J.H., Schwartz, H.L., Koerner, D., and Surks, M.I. Limited binding capacity sites for L-triiodothyronine in rat liver nuclei: Nuclear cytoplasmic interrelation binding constants and cross-reactivity with L-triiodothyronine. *J. Clin. Invest.* 1974; 53:768-777.

Ratcliffe, J.G., Stack, B.H.R., Burt, R.W., et al. Thyroid function in lung cancer. *Br. Med. J.* 1978; 1:210-212.

Redding, R.A., Douglas, W.H.J., and Stein, M. Thyroid hormone influence upon lung surfactant metabolism. *Science* 1972; 175:994-996.

Rooney, S.A., and Motoyama, I.K. (1977): Biochemical studies on normal and hormone accelerated development of pulmonary surfactant. *In: Proc. 16th Annual Hanford Biology Symp.*, ERDA, p. 162.

Rooney, S.A., Marino, P.A., Gobran, L.I., et al. Thyrotropin releasing hormone increases the amount of surfactant in lung lavage from fetal rabbits. *Pediat. Res.* 1979; 13:623-625.

Ryan, J.W., Stewart, J.M., Leary, W.P., and Ledingham, J.G. Metabolism of angiotensin 1 in the pulmonary circulation. *Biochem. J.* 1970; 120: 221-223.

Sack, J., Mashiach, S., Barkai, G., et al. Intra-amniotic thyroxine (T_4) absorption by the premature human foetus. *Acta Endocrinol.* 1979; 90:361-364.

Sakuruda, T., Milch, P.O., Lazarus, J.H., and Sterling, K. Partial purification of thyroid hormone receptor from mitochondrial inner membrane: Evidence for a physiologic role. *Trans. Assoc. Am. Physi.* 1978; 91: 403-415.

Schanker, L.S. Drug absorption from the lung. *Biochem. Pharmacol.* 1978; 27:381-385.

Schapiro, S. Metabolic and maturational effects of thyroxine on the infant rat. *Endocrinology* 1966; 78:527-532.

Schapiro, S. Some physiological, biochemical and behavioral consequences of neonatal hormone administration: Cortisol and thyroxine. *Gen. Comp. Endocrin.* 1968; 10:214-228.

Schiller, H., and Bensch, K. De novo fatty acid synthesis and elongation of fatty acids by subcellular fractions of lung. *J. Lipid. Res.* 1971; 12: 248-255.

Shinizky, M., Goldfisher, A., Bruck, A., et al. A new method for assessment of fetal lung maturity. *Br. J. Obstet. Gynaec.* 1976; 83:838-844.

Simillia, S., and Anitolainen. I. Accelerated maturity in fetal thyrotoxicosis. *Acta Paediat. Scand. Suppl.* 1970; 206:142-143.

Smith, B.T., Torday, J.S., and Giroud, C.J.P. The growth promoting effect of cortisol on human fetal lungs. *Steroids* 1973; 22:515-524.

Smith, B.T., and Torday, J.S. Factors affecting lecithin synthesis by fetal lung cells in culture. *Pediat. Res.* 1974; 8:848-851.

Smith, C.W., Bean, J.W., and Bauer, R. Thyroid influence in reactions to oxygen at atmospheric pressure. *Am. J. Physiol.* 1960; 199:883-888.

Stein, M., Kimbel, P., and Johnson, R.L. Pulmonary function in hyperthyroidism. *J. Clin. Invest.* 1961; 40:348-363.

Steinberg, H., Bassett, D., and Fisher, A. Depression of pulmonary 5-hydroxytryptamine uptake by metabolic inhibitors. *Am. J. Physiol.* 1975; 228:1298-1303

Steinberg, H., Das, D.K., Moy, W., et al. Injury to pulmonary endothelium induced by superoxide radical. *Am. Rev. Resp. Dis.* 1979; 119:364.

Steinberg, H., and Das, D.K. Competition between platelets and lung for 5-hydroxytryptamine uptake. *Exp. Lung Res.* 1980; 1:121-130.

Sterling, K., Lazarus, J.H., Milch, P.O., et al. Mitochondrial thyroid hormone receptor: Localization and physiological significance. *Science* 1978; 201:1126-1129

Stern, L. Current advances in perinatal medicine. *Paediatrician* 1979; 8(suppl. 1):76-92.

Taylor, L., and Polgar, P. Self regulation by human diploid fibroblasts via prostaglandin production. *Febs Lett.* 1977; 79:69-72.

Taylor, L., Polgar, P., McAteer, J.A., and Douglas, W.H.J. Prostaglandin production by type II alveolar epithelial cells. *Biochim. Biophys. Acta* 1979; 572:502-509.

Tsai, J.S., and Chen, A. Effect of L-triiodothyronine on $(-)^3$H-dihydro-
   alprenolol binding and cyclic AMP response to (—) adrenaline in cultured
   heart cells. *Nature* 1978; 275:138-140.
Vidik, A. Connective tissues—possible implication of the temporal changes
   for the aging process. *Mech. Aging Devel.* 1979; 9:267-285.
Wahl, L.M., Olsen, C.E., Sandberg, A.L., and Mergenhagen, S.E. Prostaglandin
   regulation of macrophage collagenase production. *Proc. Nat. Acad.
   Sci. (USA)* 1977; 74:4955-4958.
Wigglesworth, J.S. Aetiology of hyaline membrane disease. *Arch. Dis. Child.*
   1979; 54:835-837.
Williams, L.T., Lefkowitz, R.J., Watanabe, A.M., et al. Thyroid hormone
   regulation of β-adrenergic receptor number. *J. Biol. Chem.* 1977; 252:
   2787-2789.
Wilson, M., Hitchcock, K.R., Douglas, W.H., and DeLellis, R.A. Hormone and
   lung. II. *Anat. Rec.* 1979; 195:611-620.
Wu, B., Kikkawa, Y., Oyzalesi, M.M., et al. *Biol. Neonate* 1973; 22:161-168.
Yam, J., and Roberts, R.J. Pharmacological alteration of oxygen-induced lung
   toxicity. *Toxicol. Appl. Pharmacol.* 1979; 47:367-375.

6

Endocrine Functions of the Lung

RAJINDER K. CHITKARA
and
FAROQUE A. KHAN

Recent research has shown that the lungs not only participate in gas exchange, but perform an important endocrine function too. The pulmonary vascular bed is a unique system because of its position in the general circulation and its vastness. The surface area of pulmonary capillaries and the capillary endothelial cells is very large to provide the lungs with their hormonal and metabolic requirements. Although removal of vasoactive substances from the blood by the lungs has been known for sometime (Starling and Verney, 1925), it has only been during the past decade that endocrine activity of the lung is being increasingly recognized. Since the work of Vane (1969) the lungs have been variously labeled a "metabolic organ" (Said, 1969) and a "chemical filter" (Junod, 1974), and have been shown to participate not only in the metabolism of numerous biologically active substances (Junod, 1975), but to be a source as well as target of hormonal action (Said, 1972; Gillis, 1973). Substances having functions as circulating hormones pass through the pulmonary circulation unaffected, whereas those that primarily serve a local function are destroyed or are removed from the blood. In this way excessive concentration of these latter substances is prevented, and the organism is protected from their deleterious effects (Vane, 1969). Furthermore, various pharmacologic agents have been shown to influence this function of the lungs (Bakhle and Vane, 1974; Gillis et al., 1974).

The purpose of this chapter is to provide an overview of what is known pertaining to the endocrine and metabolic activity of the lung. Though most of the available data are derived from *in vitro* experiments, the clinical implications may be quite significant.

ENDOGENOUS AMINES

5-Hydroxytryptamine (5-HT; Serotonin)

5-hydroxytryptamine (serotonin) is a potent vasopressor amine. It is formed by decarboxylation of 5-hydroxytryptophan. The enzyme-decarboxylase is also present in the lung (Sadavongiwad, 1970). Conceivably, 5-HT could, therefore, be synthesized in situ in the lung. Other sources for the 5-HT pool of the lung include, the 5-HT in trapped platelets in the lungs, and the mast cells.

The pulmonary uptake of 5-HT is a saturable, energy-requiring process. The uptake sites are probably located in the endothelial cells of pulmonary capillaries (Strüm and Junod, 1972). Its transport across the cellular membrane in the pulmonary circulation is probably dependent upon the sodium-carrier system (Junod, 1972; Iwasawa et al., 1973). Hypothermia, sodium-free perfusion medium, anoxia, tricyclic antidepressants, cocaine, phenoxybenzamine, and ouabain in higher concentrations inhibit 5-HT uptake (Iwasawa et al., 1973; Junod, 1972; Alabaster and Bakhle, 1970; Gruby et al., 1971; Iwasawa and Gillis, 1974). Glucose-free perfusion medium, normetanephrine, metaraminol, reserpine, and monoamine oxidase inhibitors do not inhibit uptake of 5-HT by the lung (Iwasawa et al., 1973; Junod, 1972; Alabaster and Bakhle, 1970; Gruby et al., 1971; Iwasawa and Gillis, 1974).

5-HT taken up by the lung is rapidly metabolized. Depending upon the species, mammalian lung can inactivate or remove up to 98% of the infused 5-HT in a single passage through the pulmonary circulation (Davis and Wang, 1965). Monoamine oxidase is probably the most important enzyme involved in the pulmonary inactivation of 5-HT in many mammalian species (Thomas and Vane, 1967). However, enzymatic inactivation does not appear to be the rate-limiting step in the removal process. In humans 5-HT passes through the lung without being deaminated (Davis, 1968; Gillis et al., 1974). This probably accounts for the absence of changes in concentration of 5-hydroxyindolacetic acid in urine from patients following pneumopnectomy (Frick and Virkula, 1961). The pulmonary removal of 5-HT is also independent of platelet binding (Davis, 1968).

The removal of 5-HT from the pulmonary circulation in humans is increased after cardiopulmonary bypass and in the presence of pulmonary hypertension (Gillis et al., 1972, 1974). It is postulated that altered blood flow, or elevated intrapulmonary arterial pressure with resultant increase in back pressure, results in capillary distension and may increase functional endothelial surface area, thereby increasing the potential for 5-HT removal (Gillis et al., 1974).

To protect the body from the effects of increased circulating 5-HT, the lungs provide an effective defense. It is considered that pulmonary removal of 5-HT in humans may be related to platelet aggregation (Baumgartner and Born, 1968). In this context, control of plasma 5-HT, possibly by the lung, could represent an important element of homeostatic control, derangement of which may be linked to postoperative venous thrombosis in humans (Gruby et al., 1971). In pulmonary embolism local release of serotonin (5-HT) causes bronchoconstriction. However, here, too, inactivation by endothelium may provide an important safeguard for the systemic circulation (Fishman and Pietra, 1974).

In the "dumping syndrome," there is an increased amount of 5-HT entering portal circulation. The lungs, in combination with the liver, manage to keep the arterial concentration of 5-HT from increasing (Peskin and Miller, 1962). The potential is better realized in the metastic intestinal carcinoid syndrome where the combined removal of circulating 5-HT by the liver and lung may not suffice, thereby resulting in elevated levels of the amine in the systemic circulation. This has led to the suggestion that some symptoms of bronchial carcinoid are due to bypassing of the normal 5-HT inactivation mechanism (Sandler, 1968).

During an anaphylactic reaction large amounts of 5-HT may be released. Here, too, the lungs probably provide a protective role whereby large amounts of the mediator are prevented from entering systemic circulation, at least in some species (Eyre et al., 1973).

Norepinephrine (NE)

Unlike 5-HT, the synthesis and release of NE,* *in situ* in the lungs, have not been established. However, the lungs' participation in the metabolism of this circulating amine has been well established. It is believed that the lungs may have a regulating

---

*For an explanation of abbreviations used throughout, see the section on "Abbreviations" at the end of the chapter.

effect on the arterial blood concentrations of NE, and this may have significant clinical implications.

The pulmonary uptake of NE is both neuronal, via the sympathetic nerve endings (Iverson, 1967), and extraneuronal, via the pulmonary capillary endothelium (Hughes et al., 1969). Extraneuronal uptake is far in excess of the neuronal uptake because the sympathetic nerve endings in the lungs are far too sparse to account for the total uptake. The pulmonary uptake of NE is a saturable, carrier-mediated, temperature- and sodium-dependent process. It is inhibited by hypothermia, sodium-free perfusion medium, anoxia, ouabain, cocaine, tricyclic antidepressants, normetanephrine, and phenoxybenzamine (Iwasawa et al., 1973; Hughes et al., 1969; Nicholas et al., 1974; Alabaster and Bakhle, 1973b). Anesthesia with halothane and nitrous oxide also inhibit (Naito and Gillis, 1973), whereas some steroids may enhance NE uptake (Iwasawa and Gillis, 1973). Monoamine oxidase and catechol-o-methyl transferase inhibitors, metaraminol, propanalol, and pretreatment with 6-dydroxydopamine do not have any effect on NE uptake by the lung (Iwasawa and Gillis, 1974; Nicholas et al., 1974; Alabaster and Bakhle, 1973b).

Removal of NE from the pulmonary circulation has been known for some time (Eiseman et al., 1964; Ginn and Vane, 1968). Depending upon the species involved, and unlike 5-HT, pulmonary removal of NE is only up to 40%. The rate-limiting step in the pulmonary removal of NE is the uptake, rather than the metabolism of the amine (Iwasawa and Gillis, 1974). Norepinephrine taken up by the pulmonary capillary endothelial cells is rapidly metabolized. Metabolic degradation predominates over storage. The amine is degraded by catechol-o-methyltransferase, and deaminated by monoamine oxidase (Hughes et al., 1969). Enzyme blockers for monoamine oxidase and catechol-o-methyl transferase markedly inhibit degradation of NE, whereas uptake remains unaffected. This selective uptake and processing of NE by the lungs may have several clinical implications.

Removal of NE by human lung has been studied by means of the "systemic pressor response" (Biron et al., 1969; Boileau et al., 1972) and by measuring the blood isotope concentration (Gillis et al., 1974). Removal of NE by human lungs appears quantitatively similar to that reported in other species. As with 5-HT, removal of NE is considerably increased after cardiopulmonary bypass and in patients with pulmonary hypertension (Gillis et al., 1972, 1974), perhaps because of increased mean transit time and thus longer contact with endothelial surfaces in the pulmonary vascular bed. Removal of NE by the lung also occurs after bolus intravenous injection of the amine either to healthy subjects or to a patient undergoing cardiac catheterization (Stjärne et al., 1975).

Antihistamines interfere with the uptake and storage of NE, and this may potentiate its systemic effects. The state of the intervening lung, especially that of the endothelium, may alter the systemic vasopressor effect. In adult respiratory distress syndrome, where damage of the capillary endothelium is severe, the prospect of comparable inhibition seems reasonable (Fishman and Pietra, 1974).

What is the physiologic significance of the removal of NE from the human pulmonary vascular bed? It is believed that the lungs regulate arterial blood concentrations of NE and thereby its vasoactive properties. The increased pulmonary removal of NE in a normotensive patient after cardiopulmonary bypass may be of clinical significance. Patients who are taken off total cardiopulmonary bypass are usually given NE afterward. This may result in less NE reaching the peripheral arteriolar bed. Accordingly, use of an amine that is not removed by the lung (e.g., epinephrine) may be preferable.

Cardiac arrythmias after tricyclic antidepressants are well documented in humans (Moir, 1973). It is possible that, since tricyclic drugs inhibit pulmonary uptake of NE, the arrythmias are probably due to an increased concentration of NE reaching the coronary circulation during tricyclic drug administration.

Alpha receptor blockage is effective in restoring cardiac function in patients following cardiopulmonary bypass for open heart surgery. Pretreatment with phenoxybenzamine has been documented to prevent low cardiac output normally anticipated following cardiopulmonary bypass (Burack et al., 1972). It is possible that since phenoxybenzamine effectively inhibits pulmonary removal of NE in perfused rabbit lung (Iwasawa and Gillis, 1974), the same effect occurs in humans, and thus the concentration of NE in the left heart will be significantly increased. This probably explains the beneficial effect of pretreatment with this drug.

Adrenaline (Epinephrine), Isoprenaline, and Dopamine

Not much data are available on the handling of these endogenous amines by the lung. However, on the basis of limited evidence, it appears that human lungs. like those of the rats (Nicholas et al., 1974), have little capacity to remove significant quantities of circulating adrenaline, isoprenaline, or dopamine.

Knowledge about the lack of inactivation of adrenaline by the lung has been available for sometime (Elliot. 1905). Studies on human lung (Boileau et al., 1971) have also revealed negligible removal of adrenaline (up to 0.5%). Similar observations were made on the handling of isoprenaline (Boileau et al., 1970) by the lung in both conscious and sedated patients.

Dopamine is present in low concentrations in the lung tissue of many mammalian species, including humans. Studies have shown that dopamine also escapes pulmonary inactivation (Boileau et al., 1972).

Histamine

Histamine is one of the major mediator of anaphylaxis. It is formed by the decarboxylation of histidine. Methylhistidine inhibits the affinity of histidine decarboxylase for histidine (Reilly and Schayer, 1968), and the histamine-forming capacity is increased during anaphylaxis and decreased after treatment with steroids (Kahlson et al., 1966).

Most of the body's histamine is contained within mast cells from which mild tissue damage can readily release this amine. And, since mast cells harbor other vasoactive substances in addition to histamine, these also are often liberated simultaneously. The human lung is rich in mast cells. The lung has the capacity to synthesize histamine, since histidine decarboxylase is present in the lung tissue (Schayer, 1956). In addition, leukocytes, red cells, and platelets (in some species), which when trapped or lodged in pulmonary capillaries, may constitute the pulmonary content of the amine.

Despite the presence of enzymes capable of oxidation and methylation within the lung, histamine is not removed during its passage through the lungs (Eiseman et al., 1964). This is attributed to barriers to the free diffusion of histamine to sites of inactivation in lung tissue (Alabaster, 1977). *In vitro* studies of a specimen of lung from a single patient during surgery have also shown negligible metabolism of endogenous histamine (Lilja et al., 1960).

The release of histamine occurs mainly during (a) anaphylaxis, as exemplified by extrinsic asthma, IgE-mediated allergic reactions, and (b) during alveolar hypoxia.

ASTHMA

Histamine release from sensitized human leukocytes and from sensitized pieces of human lung have been reviewed by Lichten-

stein (1971) and Kaliner and Austen (1973). According to
Lichtenstein (1971), antigen-induced and IgE-mediated histamine
release occurs in two stages. The first is the activation stage,
which is antigen dependent and calcium independent. The second
stage is the release stage, which is antigen independent and calcium
dependent. The activation stage is under control of adenylcyclase,
stimulation of which results in decreased histamine release.
Prostaglandin E_1 (PGE_1), which, like catecholamines, stimulates
adenyl-cyclase, inhibits the activation stage. Catecholamine- (like
isoproternol) induced inhibition is markedly reduced by the beta-
blocker, propanolol, but not by the alpha-blocker, phentolamine.
Theophylline and dibutryl cyclic AMP also primarily inhibit the
activation stage, though they have a small but significant inhibitory
effect on the second or release stage as well. The second, Ca^{++}-
requiring, stage of the phenomenon is also inhibited by the
metabolic inhibitor, 2-deoxyglucose (2-DG). Diethylcarbamazine
inhibits both the activation and release stage equally. The action
of cyclic AMP active drugs early in the reaction sequence
strengthens the hypothesis that this system operates as a "second
messenger" in the allergic release of histamine (Lichtenstein and
De Bernardo, 1971).

According to Kaliner and Austen (1973), antigen activation of
human lung fragments sensitized with IgE and the release of the
chemical mediators—histamine, slow reacting substance of anaphylaxis (SRS-A)—are a sequential process.

It appears to proceed from the calcium-requiring activation of
DFP- (Di-isopropyl fluorophosphate) sensitive serine esterase;
further autocatalytic activation of the esterase; a 2-DG (2-
deoxyglucose) inhibitable energy requirement; a second Ca^{++}
requiring EDTA (ethylenediaminetetraacetate) inhibitable stage;
and a cyclic AMP inhibitable step to the release of histamine and
SRS-A (Fig. 1). Because synthesis of SRS-A involves serine esterase
and release of histamine and release of eosinophil chemotactic factor
of anaphylaxis (ECFA) and SRS-A also involves serine esterase, and
as arylsulfatase inactivates SRS-A (Orange et al., 1974; Wasserman
et al., 1975), these phenomena could modulate the release of
chemical mediators. An increase of 3', 5"-adenosine monophosphate
(cyclic AMP) by β-adrenergic agents or by a xanthine derivative
decreases histamine release; α-adrenergic agents decrease cyclic
AMP and promote an increase in mediator release. The increase
in mediator release can also occur with an increase of 3', 5'-
guanosine monophosphate (cyclic GMP) by acetylcholine or
carbachol, and is blocked by atropine (Orange et al., 1974; Kaliner
and Austen, 1974) (Fig. 2).

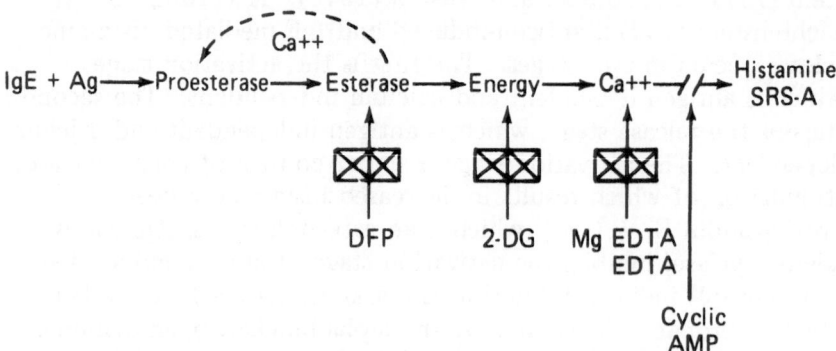

Fig. 1. The sequence of biochemical events in the antigen induced release of chemical mediators from human lung tissue sensitized with IgE. (Reprinted with permission from M. Kaliner and K.F. Austen, A sequence of biochemical events in the antigen-induced release of chemical mediators from sensitized human lung tissue, *J. Exp. Med.* 138:1077-1094, 1973.)

Finally, since intactness of microtubules in mast cells is a prerequisite for histamine and other mediator release, colchicine could block histamine release from sensitized cells. Deutrium oxide (D_2O) reverses the effect of colchicine (Gillespie and Lichtenstein, 1972).

ALVEOLAR HYPOXIA

Histamine, as the mediator released during hypoxia, has not been universally confirmed. Hass and Bergofsky (1972) in their study on rats reported a relatively high concentration of mast cells that were located near the pulmonary arteries. These mast cells were degranulated during hypoxia. Kay et al. (1974) observed an increased number of mast cells without an increased histamine-forming capacity during chronic hypoxia in rats. However, during acute hypoxia, there was no degranulation of mast cells in their study.

Acetylcholine

Lungs of various species do contain acetycholinesterases and pseudo-cholinesterases. However, inactivation of acetylcholine during its passage through the pulmonary circulation has not been established (Eiseman et al., 1964).

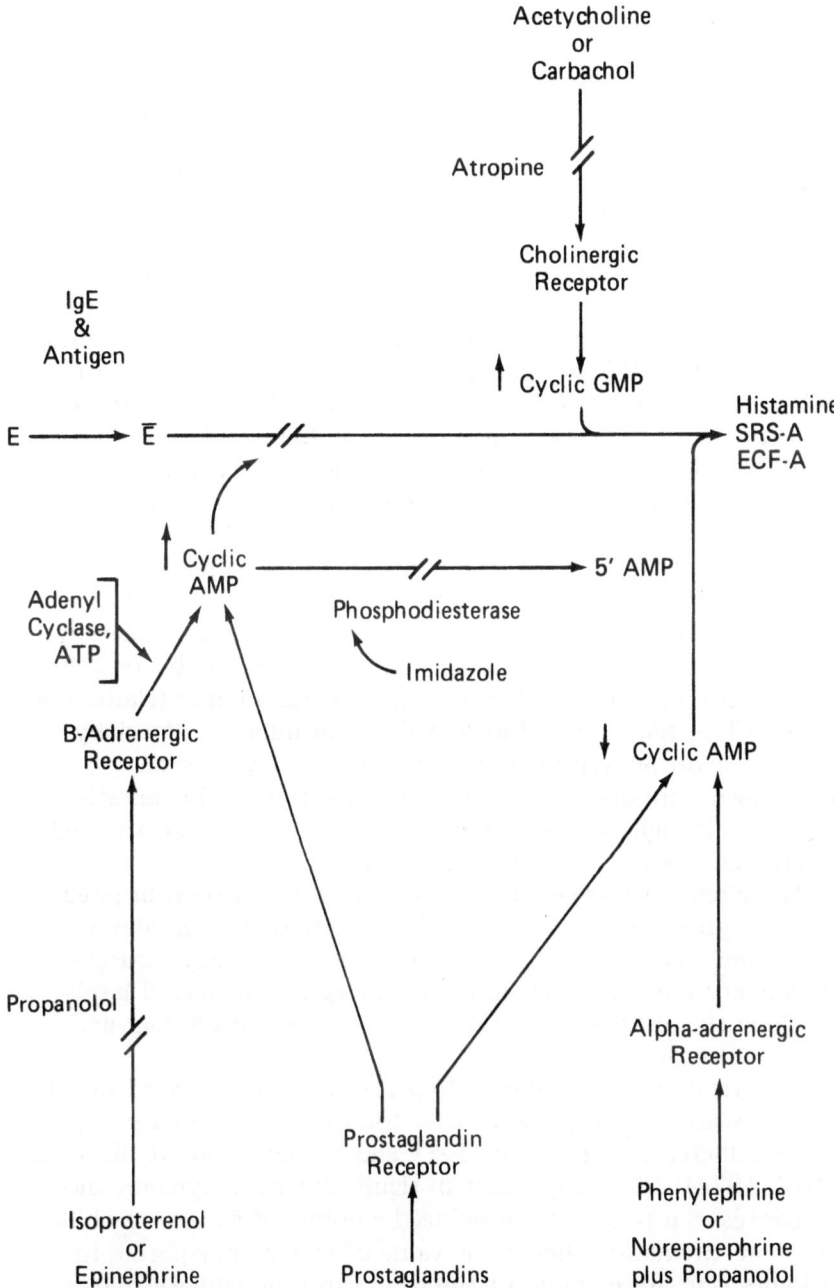

Fig. 2. Pharmacologic modulation of the antigen-induced, IgE-dependent secretion of chemical mediators from human lung tissue. E to Ē depict the series of events that precede the modulation. (Reprinted with permission from M. Kaliner and K.F. Austen, Cyclic nucleotides and modulation of effector systems of inflammation, *Biochem. Pharmacol.* 23:763–771, 1974.)

SIGNIFICANCE OF ENDOGENOUS AMINES

From the foregoing review it is evident that among the amines only 5-HT and noradrenaline are metabolized intracellularly after uptake from the plasma. Adrenaline, isoprenaline, dopamine, and acetycholine are unaffected by traversing lungs, and histamine is discharged from intrapulmonary stores into blood during anaphylaxis.

The pulmonary circulation, because of its position, blood supply, and surface area of cells comprising the alveolar capillaries, controls levels of circulating hormones reaching the arterial circulation, as is the case with 5-HT and noradrenaline. This in turn influences the cardiovascular and other responses produced by these hormones. Defects in this metabolic function of the lung could prove to be implicated in some clinical conditions, as has been observed in patients on estradiol and corticosterone therapy. These steroids inhibit removal of noradrenaline, and possibly 5-HT as well (Iwasawa and Gillis, 1973). It is possible that increased levels of circulating 5-HT could contribute to the increased risk of thrombosis during oral contraceptive and other steroid therapy.

The anesthetics, halothane and nitrous oxide, inhibit or abolish inactivation of noradrenaline in experimental animals (Naito and Gillis, 1973, Bakhle and Block, 1976). In humans, especially in surgery involving hypothermia when pulmonary removal mechanisms are depressed, halothane or nitrous oxide anesthesia may permit high concentrations of vasoactive materials to reach arterial circulation, with deleterious effects.

The circulating levels of noradrenaline are increased in pheo-chromocytoma and those of 5-HT are increased in carcinoid syndrome. The increased levels of these amines may saturate pulmonary removal mechanisms with resulting increased levels reaching the arterial circulation, thus resulting in vascular and cardiac disorders.

In patients with pulmonary hypertension secondary to valvular heart disease, and in patients after total cardiopulmonary bypass, there is increased removal of 5-HT and noradrenaline (Gillis et al., 1972, 1974). This may result in significant hemodynamic disturbances as a result of the reduced amount of amines reaching systemic circulation—hence the value of giving epinephrine to patients who are coming off the total cardiopulmonary bypass, since this amine is not inactivated by the lung.

The discharge of histamine during anaphylaxis and the resulting broncho- and vasoconstriction have already been mentioned.

The lung may also be a source of amine release in neoplasia. Bronchial adenoma and oat cell carcinoma of the lung have been shown to secrete 5-hydroxytryptophan, 5-HT, and histamine, along with peptides (kinins) and prostaglandins (Lead Article, 1968). Increased levels of 5-HT have also been reported with increased secretion of ectopic ACTH in oat cell carcinoma of the lung (Horai et al., 1973).

KININS (BRADYKININ AND RELATED PEPTIDES)

Kinins, the prototype of which is bradykinin, are a group of polypeptides with potent biologic activity (Schachter, 1964). Other polypeptides, such as oxytocin, vasopressin, eledoisin, and substance "P," have properties similar to kinins, but lack the properties kinins possess as possible chemical mediators of inflammation.

Bradykinin has potent systemic effects once it reaches the systemic arterial circulation, It causes contraction of smooth muscle and hypotension due to vasodilation; and is a mediator of inflammation. The effects of bradykinin on the pulmonary circulation are variable. It causes both an increase and a decrease in the pulmonary vasculature tone, a variability possibly related to oxygen tension and to the tone of the pulmonary vasculature at the beginning of the experiment (Konzett and Bauer, 1966; Waaler, 1961), and to the content of endogenous vasoactive substances such as catecholamines (Eltherington et al., 1968).

Kinins have been suggested as being involved in a wide variety of pathologic conditions, including carcinoid syndrome, hereditary angioneurotic oedema, pancreatitis, thermal burns, the dumping syndrome, and as part of the endogens (Collier, 1970) in clinical allergies, including asthma (other endogens being histamine, slow-reacting substance of anaphylaxis), neurologic disturbances (including migraine), arthritidies, certain transfusion reactions, protozoal infections, shock reactions [e.g., hemmorrhagic, endotoxic (Schachter, 1969)], and in the pathogenesis of emphysema (Erdös and Yang, 1970). Kinins have also been implicated in several physiologic processes, including constriction of ductus arteriosus and other circulatory changes at birth (Melmon et al., 1968) and control of airflow in the lung (Davis and Goodfriend, 1969).

The lungs have the capacity to generate as well as inactivate kinins. Blood flowing through the pulmonary circuit contains inactive precursors (kininogens). And within the substance of the lung and in the formed elements of blood are activatable kinino-

genases. Activation of the Hageman factor (Factor XII) triggers
the kinin-forming system, resulting in the formation of kallikreins
from their inactive precursors, kallikreinogen. Kallikreins cleave
kininogen, a glycoprotein (alpha 2 globulin), to effect the release
of polypeptide-kinin (Schachter, 1969) (Fig. 3).

Plasma kinins are rapidly inactivated by kinases, which act by
splitting off either the C-terminal aminoacid residue or the C-
terminal dipeptide (Said, 1973). Unlike other organs, the lungs
play a dominant role in the inactivation of bradykinin. Almost
as much as 80% of the bradykinin passing through the pulmonary
circulation is inactivated (Ferreira and Vane, 1967a). This involves
degradation by hydrolysis of the enzyme dipeptidylcarboxypeptidase. The enzyme is located in free communication with the
vascular space, probably confined to the endothelial surface (Ryan
et al., 1972; Smith and Ryan, 1972). It has been suggested that
clevage of bradykinin occurs in a microenvironment, possibly in the
pinocytic vesicles (Ryan et al., 1970).

Not all kinins are catabolized in the lung. Among bradykinin-
related substances that escape pulmonary inactivation are eledoisin,
physalaemin, and substance "P" (Boileau et al., 1970).

Many substances inhibit pulmonary bradykinase activity, thereby
potentiating the effects of bradykinin *in vivo*. BPF (bradykinin
potentiating factor), a peptide derived from snake venom, is the
most important inhibitor of bradykinase activity (Ferreira, 1965).
Not only does it inhibit bradykinin inactivation, but it also inhibits
angiotensin I conversion (Engel et al., 1972). 2-Mercaptoethanol
(2-ME) inhibits bradykinin inactivation but does not inhibit angiotensin I conversion (Stewart and Freer, 1973).

In the isolated lung, inactivation of bradykinin is prevented by
venom peptides and BAL (2:3 dimercaptopropanol), but not by
2-ME (Alabaster and Bakhle, 1973a) despite its ability to potentiate the effects of bradykinin *in vivo* (Scholz and Biron, 1969).
In lung homogenates, both the crude particulate bradykinase and
the highly purified dipeptidylcarboxypeptidases of the lung
hydrolize bradykinin and convert angiotensin I to angiotensin II.
They are inhibited by chelating agents (such as EDTA and BAL),
snake venom peptides, other peptides such as B-chain of insulin,
and angiotensin I. The enzymatic activity is chloride dependent
and its pH optimum is between 7 and 8 (Alabaster and Bakhle,
1973a; Alabaster and Bakhle, 1972a,b; Igic et al., 1972).

Other than dipeptidylcarboxypeptidases, lung homogenates also
contain aminopeptidase and endopeptidase. However, these kinases
remain to be investigated. It is speculated than an endopeptidase
in the presence of Borthrops peptidase inhibitors may also inactivate
bradykinin quite rapidly (Ferreira and Bakhle, 1977).

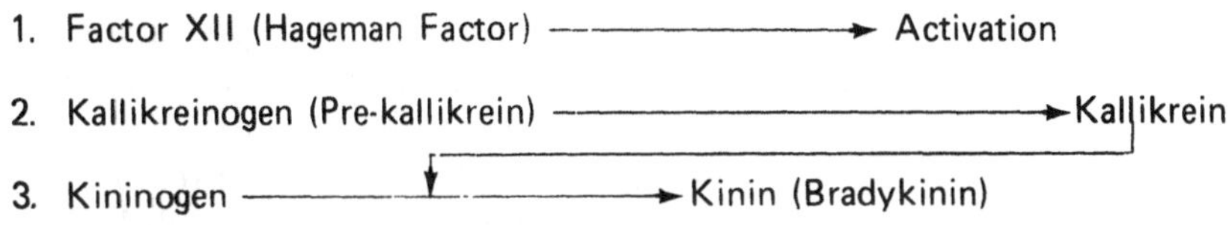

1. Factor XII (Hageman Factor) ────────────→ Activation

2. Kallikreinogen (Pre-kallikrein) ──────────────→Kallikrein

3. Kininogen ─────────┴─────────→ Kinin (Bradykinin)

Fig. 3. Activation of Hageman factor in the lung.

Though lung homogenates contain other metabolizing enzymes, mention may be made of the divergence in the metabolic activity of lung *in vivo* and *in vitro* that has been observed. Lung homogenates readily inactivate histamine, although histamine is unaffected by passage through the pulmonary vascular bed (Boileau et al., 1970; Bakhle and Vane, 1974). Other evidence of divergence is noted with angiotensin II, which is unaffected during its passage through the vascular bed (Goffinet and Murlow, 1965; Biron et al., 1969), though the lung homogenates have been shown to have angiotensinase activity. Eledoisin, a kinin-like hypotensive peptide, is another example of divergence between *in vitro* and *in vivo* conditions. This peptide, though resistant to plasma kinases, is metabolized by lung homogenates, but is unaffected during its passage through the pulmonary vascular bed (Ferreira and Vane, 1967a).

Substance "P"

Substance "P" is a hypotensive peptide. It is present in the central nervous system and in the intestinal mucosa. It escapes pulmonary inactivation (Boileau et al., 1970; Stewart, 1971), but is degraded by thromboplastin, as has been shown *in vitro* studies (Simmons et al., 1974).

The fact that it is unaffected during its passage through the pulmonary circulation argues for it to have a role as a circulating hormone (Stewart, 1971).

Angiotensin

Renin, an enzyme present in the juxtaglomerular apparatus of the kidney, acts on the renin substrate—an α-2-globulin known as angiotensinogen—to form angiotensin I, which is a decapeptide. This is a relatively inactive pressor agent. Angiotensin I is, in turn, acted on by the converting enzyme to form angiotensin II, which is an octapeptide. The converting enzymes activity is present in the plasma, lungs, kidney, etc. (Skeggs et al., 1956; Ng and Vane, 1970; Ryan et al., 1972; Fishman and Pietra, 1974) and is a dipeptidylcarboxypeptidase. Angiotensin II is a potent pressor agent whose activity is terminated by angiotensinases, which have a wide tissue distribution (Ledingham and Leary, 1974) (Fig. 4).

The presence of the converting enzyme in the plasma has been known for some time (Skeggs et al., 1956). But the activity of the converting enzyme is too low to account for the rapid conversion of angiotensin I or II (Fishman and Pietra, 1974). Since the observation that angiotensin II passed through the pulmonary vascular bed unchanged (Goffinet and Murlow, 1965; Ng and Vane, 1967) and that the conversion of angiotensin I to II in the blood was slow (17% after 30 seconds), whereas the conversion in the pulmonary circulation was rapid (40–50% in less than 10 seconds) (Ng and Vane, 1967), considerable insight has been gained in the activation process of angiotensin I. Recent research has shown that the lung contains angiotensin I converting enzyme, which, like the one in the plasma, is a dipeptidase; that the pulmonary conversion is indeed the most important physiologically; and that the activation/inactivation by the blood is relatively unimportant (Ng and Vane, 1970; Oparil et al., 1971; Ryan et al., 1972; Osborn et al., 1972). The only species difference is in rats, where extrapulmonary conversion of angiotensin I to II is very significant and no pulmonary conversion occurs, even though bradykinin is up to 95% inactivated (Freer and Stewart, 1975).

The pulmonary angiotensin-converting enzyme (dipeptide hydrolase) has been isolated by several investigators (Bakhle et al., 1969; Huggins et al., 1970; Oparil et al., 1971; Igic et al., 1972; Soffer et al., 1974). The enzyme is a glycoprotein with a single polypeptide chain and a molecular weight of approximately 136,000 daltons. The carbohydrate content of the enzyme is about 16% and contains galactose, N-acetylglucosamine, and mannose. Its pH optima vary, depending upon the substrate used. However, the activity of the enzyme is chloride dependent (Cushman and Cheung, 1971; Doser et al., 1972; Igic et al., 1972; Yang et al., 1971; Sandler et al., 1971). The activity of the converting enzyme, though not universal, has been reported to be inhibited by chelating agents such as EDTA (ethylene diamino-tetraacetic acid) and BAL (dimercaprol), heavy metal ions, and 2-mercaptoethanol. Inhibition has also been observed in the presence of peptides, such as insulin and its B-chain, bradykinin, and snake venom peptides, such as BPF (Bakhle, 1971; Ondetti et al., 1971).

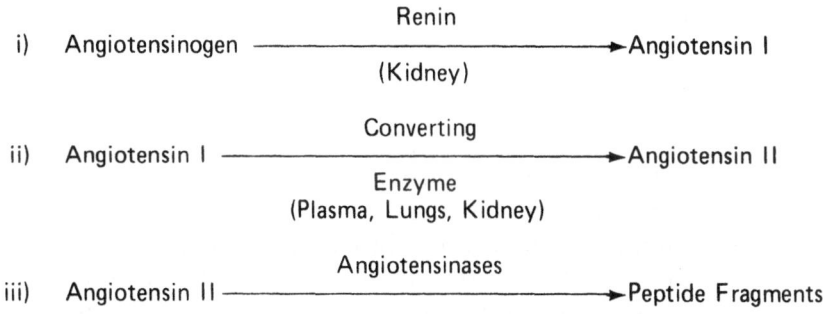

Fig. 4. Metabolism of angiotensin.

The pulmonary angiotensin-converting enzyme is located on the endothelial surface (Soffer et al., 1974; Ryan et al., 1972) and is directly accessible to the blood flowing through the lungs (Ryan et al., 1972). The subcellular localization has been further documented by the use of a marker-tagged antibody to pig lung converting enzyme (Ryan et al., 1975, 1976). Caldwell et al. (1976), using a fluorescein-tagged converting enzyme antibody, have demonstrated the presence of converting enzyme in the luminal cells. The high carbohydrate content also favors the conclusion that the enzyme is a membrane protein and part of the endothelial structure (Soffer et al., 1974).

The C-terminal structure of angiotensin I (Fig. 5) is a prerequisite for the activation of the angiotensin converting enzyme (Oparil et al., 1971; Soffer et al., 1974). Activation in the lungs involves cleavage of histidine and leucine from the C-terminal of angiotensin I. Some extrapulmonary conversion (e.g., in kidneys and hind limbs) of angiotensin I to II also occurs (Favre et al., 1974). However, unlike the lungs, these organs are more concerned with inactivating rather than generating angiotensin II. This disparate behavior of the lungs and systemic circulation may have to do with its anatomical location (membrane surface in lung versus intracellular in systemic vascular endothelium) and hence the accessibility (Bakhle et al., 1969).

Relationship Between Pulmonary Metabolism of Angiotensin and Bradykinin

Both angiotensin and bradykinin are potent peptides with opposite effects on the blood pressure. Evidence is now convincing that the pulmonary angiotensin-converting enzyme is identical with

H_2N - Asp - Arg - Val - Tyr - Ile - His - Pro - Phe - His - Leu - COOH

Fig. 5. Angiotensin I structure.

kininase, which inactivates bradykinin. The evidence is based on
the following observations (Said, 1973):

1. Both bradykinin and angiotensin I disappear almost completely in a single circulation through the lungs.
2. Factors that potentiate the action of bradykinin (BPF-like
   peptides from snake venom) also inhibit the angiotensin I
   converting enzyme (Soffer et al., 1974).
3. Both the conversion of angiotensin I to II and the inactivation of bradykinin involve the splitting off of the C-terminal
   dipeptide which is His-Leu for angiotensin I and Phe-Arg
   for bradykinin (Alabaster and Bakhle, 1972; Igic et al., 1972)
   (Fig. 6).
4. The enzyme, dipeptide hydrolase (Igic et al., 1972), is an
   angiotensin-converting enzyme and a kinase. In other words,
   while angiotensin I is converted to the more potent angiotensin II, bradykinin is inactivated, and neither the hormone
   nor its metabolic products are retained by the lungs (Ryan
   et al., 1972).
5. Both angiotensin I conversion and bradykinin inactivation
   apparently take place in the plasma membrane and pinocytic
   vesicles of the capillary endothelial cells where there is ready
   accessibility to the enzyme, dipeptide hydrolase (Ryan et al.,
   1972).

Clinical Significance of Pulmonary Angiotensin Converting Enzyme

The physiologic significance of the pulmonary conversion of
angiotensin I is uncertain. Converting enzyme, responsible for
hydrolysis of angiotensin I to II, has been demonstrated in the
human lung (Fritz and Overturf, 1972; Overturf et al., 1975).
Despite the lack of direct evidence, it has nevertheless been
generally assumed that angiotensin I is converted to angiotensin II
in human lung, as it is in the lungs of experimental animals
(Bakhle and Vane, 1974). Furthermore, inhibitors of the converting enzyme, as demonstrated in experimental animals, act in
humans also, and one such inhibitor is a nonapeptide designated
SQ 20881 (Collier et al., 1973). This substance has been shown to
cause a significant and prolonged reduction of blood pressure in

a)   Angiotensin I

   H_2N - Asp - Arg - Val - Tyr - Ile - His - Pro - Phe - <u>His - Leu - COOH</u>

b)   Bradykinin

   H_2N - Arg - Pro - Pro - Gly - Phe - Ser - Pro - <u>Phe - Arg - COOH</u>

Fig. 6. Angiotensin I and bradykinin structure.

12 of 13 patients tested (Gavras et al., 1974). Though these data do not necessarily prove that inhibition of lung-converting enzyme is the cause of altered pressor response to angiotensin I, they may be a pointer to the potential usefulness of the competitive inhibitors that will block conversion of angiotensin I to II in high renin hypertension.

The biologic paradox of angiotensin (pressor amine) activation and bradykinin (depressor) inactivation by the dipeptidase in the regulation of blood pressure is intriguing. It is possible that lungs regulate the blood pressure not only by controlling the angiotensin I conversion and bradykinin inactivation, but also by liberating prostaglandins (Zusman et al., 1974) and histamine.

Angiotensin II

Angiotensin II, an octapeptide, escapes pulmonary removal and inactivation in humans (Biron et al., 1969) and in other mammalian species (Bakhle and Vane, 1974), thereby substantiating its role as a circulating hormone.

EOSINOPHIL CHEMOTACTIC FACTOR OF ANAPHYLAXIS (ECFA)

ECFA is an acidic peptide of low molecular weight (approximately 500 daltons) (Austen, 1974). Like histamine, it is stored preformed in mast cell granules (Wasserman et al., 1974a).

Release of ECFA, along with histamine and SRS-A, has been demonstrated *in vitro* from the human lung and the lungs of many species (Kay et al., 1971). The conditions necessary for the release of ECFA are an intact glycolytic pathway, divalent cations, and DFP-sensitive esterase. Cyclic nucleotides modify the release

of ECFA in a manner similar to that with histamine and SRS-A
(Wasserman et al., 1974b). Disodium cromoglycate probably also
inhibits the release of ECFA from human lung (Kaliner and
Austen, 1974).

ECFA is selectively chemotactic toward eosinophils that are
rich in arylsulfatase. Since arylsulfatase inactivates SRS-A (Orange
et al., 1975), release of ECFA may be an example of a feedback
mechanism occurring in the lung during anaphylaxis.

OTHER PEPTIDES

Vasopressin (ADH) and oxytocin activities are unaffected during
their passage through the lung. The role of the lung in the
handling of gastrin is uncertain. However, a small amount of
insulin is lost during its passage through the lung (Rubenstein et al.,
1968).

Polypeptide Hormones (Ectopic Hormone Syndromes)

The lung may be an important endocrine organ in disease. The
production of polypeptide hormones, resulting in "ectopic hormone
syndromes," has been known for some time (Knowles and Smith,
1960), and is of considerable clinical and biochemical significance.
Ectopic endocrine syndromes occur most often with bronchogenic
carcinoma, but have also been reported in nonmalignant conditions
(Bryant, 1972). These syndromes may manifest individually or in
combination, as is often the case with anaplastic cell carcinoma of
the lung.

Only a brief description of the polypeptide hormone secretion
in pulmonary disease, the resultant syndrome, and commonly
associated lesions will be presented to emphasize the role of lung
as a source of hormones.

Endocrinopathies account for approximately 10% of all cases
of bronchogenic carcinoma (Said, 1974). The most common are
due to parathormone or related polypeptides (PTH), adreno-
corticotrophic hormone (ACTH), and antiduiretic hormone (ADH).

ACTH Secretion

Excessive secretion of this hormone results in hypokalemic
alkalosis, edema. and Cushing's syndrome. The hypokalemia,

weakness, impaired glucose tolerance, edema, and hypertension are due to hypercortisolism. Signs of Cushing's syndrome, such as centripetal obesity, cutaneous striae, and osteoporosis, take longer to develop and appear only with slowly growing malignancies (Liddle et al., 1965). Oat cell carcinoma is the most common associated lesion, but the syndrome has also been reported with bronchial adenoma and adenocarcinoma of the lung (Poole et al., 1970; Sachs et al., 1970).

Rarely in patients with ectopic ACTH secretion is evidence for the presence of other peptides such as the corticotropin-releasing factor (CRF) (Upton and Amatrudda, 1971), melanocyte-stimulating hormone (MSH) (Omen, 1970), and amines such as serotonin (Horai et al., 1973) may be present, whereas other peptides such as ADH may be suppressed (Davidson, 1972).

The elevated ACTH levels are not suppressible with dexamethasone. Assaying plasma and even bronchial washings for immunoreactive "big" ACTH have been stressed and may serve not only as a marker in the diagnosis of bronchogenic carcinoma, but also as a predictor of prognosis, as high levels of this hormone correlate with short survival times (Ayvazian et al., 1975). Also, plasma levels of corticosteroids usually rise with dissemination of the disease and fall after removal of the primary lesion.

Inappropriate Secretion of Antidiuretic Hormone (ADH)

Inappropriate secretion of ADH occurs most commonly with oat cell carcinoma. However, the syndrome has also been reported with bronchial adenoma; adenocarcinoma; alveolar cell carcinoma; pulmonary infections, including tuberculosis, aspergillosis, staphylococcal, and influenzal pneumonia and lung abscess (Barter, 1973; Rosenow et al., 1972; Bryant, 1972; Spanos and Spry, 1974).

Patients with this syndrome have hyponatremia, their urine osmolality exceeding that of plasma in the presence of normal renal and adrenal function (Barter, 1973). The qualification "inappropriate" applied to ADH secretion relates to the fact that secretion continues despite reduction in plasma osmolality. This, in turn, because of increased circulating volume, results in decreased aldosterone secretion. Because of increased ADH and reduced aldosterone secretion, the resultant hyponatremia is both diluting and depletive (Ross, 1963).

Bioassay has shown increased levels of ADH (arginine-vasopressin) in urine and plasma, as well as in extracts of neoplasms, and in tuberculous lung tissue of patients with this syndrome.

Bronchogenic tumors have also been demonstrated to synthesize vasopressin *in vitro* (Said, 1974).

Hyperparathyroidism

Hypercalemia associated with bronchogenic carcinoma, and without bony metastases, is most commonly due to the secretion of parathormone (PTH) or related peptide (Roof et al., 1971; Reiss, 1974). The syndrome has been reported with squamous cell carcinoma, adenocarcinoma, and large cell anaplastic carcinoma, as well as with sarcomas, lymphomas, and leukemias. Hypercalcemia is also a recognized complication of sarcoidosis (Winnacker et al., 1968).

Patients with this syndrome (usually when serum calcium values reach 15–17 mg%) have drowsiness, hypotonia, polyuria, poly-dypsia. irritability, constipation, and abdominal pain. Semicoma or coma may develop mimicking brain metastases (Taylor and Siemsen, 1965).

It has been suggested (Roof et al., 1971) that the ectopic syndrome is associated with two or more types of parathyroid hormone, one identical to the secretion of parathyroid gland, and another of different immunogenecity. This may help, in some cases, in the differential diagnosis of ectopic from primary hyperparathyroidism.

Gonadotropin Secretion

Increased gonadotropin levels in the blood, urine, and neoplastic tissue have been found in patients with a wide variety of carcinomas of the lung, including large cell anaplastic carcinoma (Dailey and Marcuse, 1969; Cotrell et al., 1969). Clinically, in children it presents with precocious puberty (Omen, 1971) and in adults with gynecomastia, which may be unilateral, and often on the side of the pulmonary lesion (Sbar, 1972). The various types of gonadotropins reported in lung tumors are luteinizing hormone (LH), follicle-stimulating hormone (FSH), human chorionic gonadotropin (HCG), and human placental lactogen (HPL) (Rosen and Weintraub, 1969).

Growth Hormone (HGH)

The syndrome of hypertrophic periosteopathy may come to

resemble acromegaly (Knowles and Smith, 1960) and occurs in patients with bronchogenic carcinoma of the squamous cell type.

The mechanism of production of this syndrome has been poorly understood. However, in some cases an increase in plasma level of growth hormone has been reported, with a return to normal levels of the hormone and disappearance of the symptoms of periosteopathy after resection of tumor (Steiner et al., 1968). Increased levels of HGH have been found in extracts of bronchogenic tumors (Beck and Burger, 1972), and synthesis of the hormone has also been demonstrated from lung carcinoma in cell culture (Greenberg et al., 1972).

Carcinoid Syndrome

Carcinoid syndrome is more commonly seen with bronchial adenoma than with bronchogenic carcinoma of the oat cell type. The tumors secrete predominantly 5-hydroxytryptophan as well as 5-HT. However, other mediators of the carcinoid syndrome may include histamine, kallikreins, kinins, other peptides, and prostaglandins (Leading Article, 1968).

In bronchial carcinoids, the signs and symptoms are usually the result of increased secretion of the amines, and at least in part to the release of kinins. The major clinical profile includes cutaneous flushing, increased lacrimation and salivation, tachycardia, and a predominence of left-sided cardiac lesions (Melmon et al., 1965).

Insulin-Like Secretion

Mesenchymal tumors of the chest secrete insulin-like peptide or insulin and may cause hypoglycemia (Omen, 1971). However, one case has been reported in the literature in which hypoglycemia was associated with squamous cell carcinoma and was relieved by removal of the primary neoplasm (Daughtry et al., 1967).

Glucagon or Related Peptide

There is one case report of fibrosarcoma of the lung associated with diabetes mellitus, with return of normoglycemia after surgical removal of the tumor (Turner and Horne, 1970). Immunoassay, revealing the presence of both insulin and glucagon from the metastases of bronchogenic carcinoma, has also been reported (Unger et al., 1964)

Prolactin

Increased prolactin secretion resulting in galactorrhoea or without any symptom has been reported with anaplastic cell carcinoma and in sarcoidosis (Turkington, 1971, 1972).

Calcitonin

Elevated levels of calcitonin have been reported in small cells and in adenocarcinoma of the lung (Silva et al., 1976). Both thyroidal and ectopic secretion of the hormone may occur, and the levels of the hormone may be a useful indicator in the follow-up of patients with bronchogenic carcinoma (Silva et al., 1976; Williams, 1976).

Vasoactive Lung Polypeptides

Normal lungs have been found to contain at least two vasoactive polypeptides (Said et al., 1975). Both dilate systemic and pulmonary vessels but have the opposite effect on extravascular smooth muscles. The chemical identity of these peptides has not been determined as yet, but a cross-immunoreactivity between the relaxant lung polypeptide fraction and vasoactive intestinal poly-peptide (VIP) has been observed (Said and Mutt, 1970). The vasoactive lung polypeptide passes through the lung unchanged.

The role of these peptides in pathologic states has not been established, although evidence for the presence of the spasmogenic lung peptide has been documented in foam and perfusates from edematous cat lungs (Said, 1977). It is also postulated that the spasmogenic lung polypeptide is one of the mediator in hypoxic pulmonary hypertension (Said et al., 1975), the others being 5-HT, histamine, and prostaglandin-like compounds. VIP or related peptide has also been found in patients with bronchogenic carcinoma who present no endocrine manifestations (Said, 1977), and may be an important tool for the detection and follow-up of lung cancer.

CELLULAR ORIGIN OF HORMONE-PRODUCING TUMORS

Hormone-producing tumors could develop in any organ that contains cells originating in primitive neural crest. Such cells have been demonstrated throughout the alimentary tract and in foregut organs, including bronchi, and have been termed as "APUD" or amine precursor uptake and decarboxylation cells (Weichert, 1970; Pearse and Polak, 1971).

These cells can concentrate and decarboxylate precursors of biogenic amines and produce polypeptide hormones, and, in neoplasia, increase their secretion, thus resulting in endocrinopathies (Weichert, 1970; Pearse and Polak, 1971).

Miscellaneous

Amylase, eosinophil chemotactic factor of anaphylaxis, placental alkaline phosphatase, and carcinoembryonic antigen are the group of peptides that have been demonstrated to be synthesized by lung tumor cells in patients with primary or metastatic lung cancer and found elevated in the sera of patients with lung cancer. Mention may also be made of the lipids, especially prostaglandins E_2 and F_2, that have also been demonstrated to be synthesized by lung tumor cells in patients with lung cancer (Robin, 1978).

Renally Active Lung Substance (LS)

This is believed to be a peptide that promotes sodium and water retention, without affecting total renal blood flow. It has been demonstrated in the lung tissue and in the arterial blood. It is thought to be formed by the action of lung on a plasma globulin (Lockett, 1972).

In conclusion, among the peptides bradykinin is inactivated, and angiotensin activated, in the pulmonary capillary bed. The metabolism of these peptides occurs at the endothelial surface. The lung has the capacity to discharge kallikreins from intra-pulmonary stores into the blood. Other peptides, such as angiotensin II, vasopressin, oxytocin, vasoactive intestinal polypeptides, and bradykinin-related substances (eledoisin, physalaemin, substance "P") are unaffected during their passage through the lungs. The fate of gastrin and insulin is uncertain, although some loss of activity of the latter during its passage through the lungs has been reported.

The lungs have also been shown to release kinins during anaphylaxis, and other polypeptides such as ACTH, ADH, and other polypeptide hormones in various diseased states.

PROSTAGLANDINS (PGs)

Prostaglandins are a group of hormones with a bewildering spectrum of biologic activity. Since their discovery by Von Euler (1934), the literature on this family of lipid acids has increased at a prodigious rate and several reviews are worthy of perusal (Bergstrom et al., 1968; Horton, 1969; Hinman, 1972; Weeks, 1972; Flower, 1974; Marrazzi and Anderson, 1974). The purpose of this review is to provide an overview of the prostaglandin metabolism by the lung.

Chemistry

Prostaglandins (PGs) are 20-carbon, unsaturated fatty acids, which have in common a cyclopentane ring and two aliphatic side chains. All have a hydroxyl group in the C-15 position, which is a key position of the molecule in terms of its effect on smooth muscle tone (Anderson and Ramwell, 1974). The parent compound is prostanoic acid (Fig. 7).

On the basis of modifications of the cyclopentane ring, several groups of PGs have been distinguished (e.g., E, F, A). The constituents of each of these groups is identified by a subscript number that refers to the number of unsaturated bonds in the aliphatic side chains; for example, E_1 has one double bond and E_2 has two double bonds.

The prostaglandins are rather ubiquitous substances and are synthesized by an enzyme complex referred to as prostaglandin synthetase (PG-synthetase). This enzyme complex appears to be present in every mammalian tissue so far investigated, as well as in several nonmammalian tissues (Horton, 1969).

The lungs contain a relative abundance of PG-synthetase. Synthesis of prostaglandins may be initiated by both physiologic and pathologic provocation. Human lungs contain 10 to 20 times more PGF_2 alpha than PGE_2, while in the bronchi PGE_2 levels are greater than PGF alpha in the ratio of 2 to 3:1. No PGE_1 or PGF alpha has been found in the human lung (Karim et al., 1967).

Prostaglandins are synthesized from essential fatty acids. The microsomal enzyme, PG-synthetase, has been isolated from guinea pig lungs (Anggard and Samuelsson, 1965). Through a sequence of oxidation and hydroxylation–cyclization an endoperoxide intermediate is formed that is subsequently transformed into PGE_2 by an enzyme endoperoxide-isomerase, and into PGF_2 alpha by an

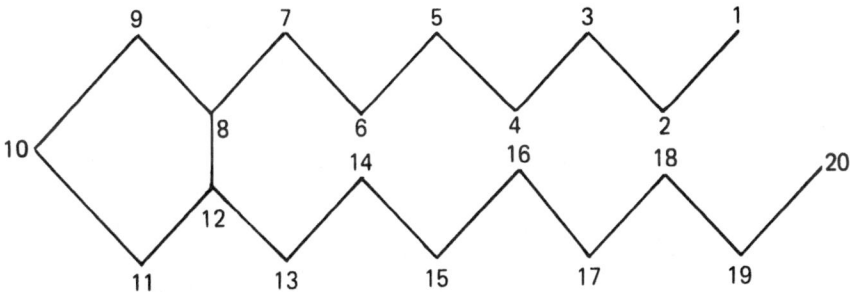

Fig. 7. Prostanoic acid.

enzyme endoperoxide reductase (Hamberg and Samuelsson, 1973). The endoperoxide intermediate has a strong biologic activity and could contract the rabbit aorta. Parkes and Eling (1974), in their studies of the PG-synthetase system in guinea pig lungs, not only found evidence for formation of predominently PGF_2 alpha, but also an unidentified PG-like compound, which may have been prostaglandin D_2.

Once formed, prostaglandins are not stored. Diverse stimuli have been shown to release prostaglandins from the lungs. Pharmacologic agents that can provoke increases in *de novo* synthesis and release include histamine, bradykinin, serotonin, and phospholipase-A (Piper, 1973a,b). In the experiments of Parkes and Eling (1974), prostaglandin synthesis was stimulated by addition of hydroxy-quinone, epinephrine, norepinephrine, and serotonin. Furthermore, serotonin seemed to favor PGF_2 alpha synthesis, whereas norepinephrine primarily stimulated the unidentified PG-like compound.

Among the mechanical and chemical stimuli shown to release prostaglandins from the lungs should be included inflation in the guinea pig (Berry et al., 1971) and dog (Said, 1973); air and particle embolization in cat (Lindsey and Wyllie, 1970) and guinea pig (Piper and Vane, 1971); anaphylaxis in sensitized guinea pig (Piper and Vane, 1969) and *in vitro* human lung preparations (Piper, 1973). It is possible that prostaglandins are released secondarily to the liberation of histamine and slow-reacting substance of anaphylaxis (Liebeg et al., 1974). Alveolar hypoxia (Said et al., 1974); pulmonary edema (Said and Yoshida, 1974); lack of ascorbic acid (Puglisi et al., 1976), and adenosine-triphosphate (Needleman et al., 1974); have also been reported to stimulate release of prostaglandins, predominently of the F type.

Certain modulations of the prostaglandins are possible. Prosta-glandin E can be dehydrated by weak alkali to form prostaglandin

A or B, and prostaglandin E can be reduced to prostaglandins of
the F series (Fanburg, 1973). It is possible that altering the rate
of production of certain prostaglandins could modify the final
biologic effect.

Many compounds are known to block the PG-synthetase activity,
and thereby inhibit the release of prostaglandins (Flower, 1974);
the most significant of are the aspirin-like drugs. Vane (1971)
observed this phenomenon in cell-free homogenates of guinea pig
lung. Since then, there have been many reports of cases in which,
regardless of the nature of stimulus—mechanical, chemical, or
immunologic, the release of prostaglandins and rabbit aorta
contracting substance (RCS) has been abolished in isolated,
perfused, or chopped lungs by aspirin-like drugs (Palmer et al.,
1970; Palmer et al., 1973; Fjalland, 1974).

It is estimated that the daily production of prostaglandin E_1
and E_2 in humans is approximately 50 to 350 μg in males and
20 to 40 μg in females (Hamberg and Samuelsson, 1971). However,
the levels of prostaglandins in plasma are reported to be very low
and are in concentrations of 50 pg/ml for E-type prostaglandins
and 10 pg/ml for PGF_2 alpha (Dray and Charbonnel, 1974). This
would suggest rapid degradation of prostaglandins. Ferreira and
Vane (1967) found that up to almost 92% of circulating
prostaglandin E_1, E_2, and F_2 alpha was inactivated during a single
passage through the lungs, whereas prostaglandins A_1 and A_2, at
least in cats and dogs, remains largely unaffected (McGiff et al.,
1967).

The lungs are a rich source of prostaglandin-catabolizing enzymes
and the pulmonary vascular bed appears to be a major site in this
respect for the metabolism of blood-borne prostaglandins. The
lungs of experimental animals contain a specific enzyme, 15-
hydroxy-PG-dehydrogenase (Anggard and Samuelsson, 1967).
The concentration of this enzyme in the lung is surpassed only by
that in the kidney and spleen. It is a NAD+ dependent enzyme,
with a pH optimum of 8.5-9 and a molecular weight of 60-70
$\times 10^3$ daltons. It is presumably a soluble cytoplasmic enzyme
(Anggard, 1971). This enzyme is responsible for the oxidation and
inactivation of prostaglandins, especially of the E and F series,
whereas prostaglandin A is less susceptible to oxidation (Bakhle
and Vane, 1974). Evidence is now available that human lungs also
biodegrade prostaglandins (Golub et al., 1975; Jose et al., 1976),
except PGA_1, which escapes biodegradation in the lung (Golub et
al., 1975).

Hamberg and Samuelsson (1971) have investigated the sequence
of reactions for the catabolism for PGE_2 in man. The initial rapid

step is the oxidation for the C-15 hydroxyl group by PG-dehydrogenase, whence prostaglandins lose most of their biologic activity. The 15-ketocompound formed is then reduced under the action of Δ^{13} reductase to give rise to a 13, 14-dihydrocompound. A similar pathway exists for PGF_2 alpha catabolism in the guinea pig lung (Granstrom, 1971).

The substrate specificity of prostaglandin dehydrogenase is greater for PGEs than the PGFs. The extent of removal of a particular series of prostaglandins has been attributed to the magnitude of dehydrogenase activity of the lung in these substrates (Samuelsson et al., 1971). This is borne out by *in vitro* studies with a swine lung preparation (Anggard and Samuelsson, 1967) and *in vivo* results obtained in dogs (McGiff et al., 1967) and in humans (Golub et al., 1975; Jose et al., 1976).

Inhibition of prostaglandin inactivation has been observed with polyphloretin phosphate as well as with diphloretin phosphate (DPP), and by sulphydryl binding agents such as sodium-p-chloromercuriphenylsulphonate and N-ethylmaleimide (Crutchley and Piper, 1974). Polyphloretin phosphate, however, has no effect on the pulmonary inactivation of bradykinin or serotonin in the isolated guinea pig lung (Crutchley and Piper, 1974). Disease processes involving the pulmonary parenchyma may also inhibit prostaglandin catabolism. This has been observed in a patient with primary pulmonary hypertension, where there was no loss of PGF_2 alpha in the pulmonary circulation (Jose et al., 1976).

Physiologic Effects of Prostaglandins in the Lungs

The major physiologic effect of prostaglandins relevant to lung is their ability to alter the smooth muscle tone of both the bronchial and vascular musculature. Current evidence suggests that PGF_2 alpha is a potent constrictor and prostaglandin E causes relaxation of the smooth muscle. Further, it has been shown that whereas PGE_1 exerts a consistent and significant broncho-dilatory action, the bronchodilator effects of PGE_2 are smaller and bronchoconstriction has been observed in several studies. However, prostaglandins of A-series have significant effects on the cardiovascular and renal systems and inconsistant stimulating effects on the airways and pulmonary vasculature, whereas those of the B-series have an inhibitory action on airways and pulmonary vasculature (Kadowitz et al., 1975).

Studies in humans (Cuthbert, 1969; Fishburne et al., 1972; Smith and Cuthbert, 1972; Mathé et al., 1973; Kamakami et al.,

1973) have shown that prostaglandins have more potent effects on
the tone of airways when given by aerosols than when intravenously
administered. This may be a reflection of the role of the pulmonary
vascular bed on the metabolism of prostaglandins. Aerosilized
PGEs are bronchodilators in asthmatic subjects (Cutbert, 1969)
and the potency of PGE_2 is greater than that of PGE_1. This may
be due to less upper airway irritation and reflex bronchoconstriction by PGE_2 (Kamakami et al., 1973). Aerosilized PGF_2 alpha
induces bronchoconstriction in both normal and asthmatic subjects.
However, the degree of bronchoconstriction is greater, and lasts
longer, in the asthmatic subjects (Mathé et al., 1973).

The response of the pulmonary vascular smooth muscle to
prostaglandins is similar to that observed in the airways. In dogs,
PGE_1 dilates and PGF_2 alpha constricts pulmonary arteries and
veins (Brody and Kadowitz, 1974). Pulmonary arterial constriction
secondary to local hypoxia is reversed by PGE_1 (Goldzimer et al.,
1974). In normal human subjects, PGE_1 induces a slight decrease
in pulmonary vascular resistance (Carlson et al., 1969).

MECHANISM OF ACTION OF PROSTAGLANDINS
ON SMOOTH MUSCLE

Current evidence suggests that prostaglandins have a direct effect
on the smooth muscle. The precise mechanism at the cellular level
is not known, but it is believed that it centers on two systems—
the adenylcyclase system and the calcium-mediated coupling of
excitation and contraction of smooth muscle.

Cyclic AMP (adenosine $3':5'$-cyclic monophosphate) is thought
to be the central intracellular mediator in tissue responses to many
hormones. Current thinking is that adenylcyclase is stimulated
by the action of hormones on target tissues to catalyze the conversion of ATP to cyclic AMP, which, in turn, causes tissues to
perform their function. Cyclic AMP is degraded by phospho-
diesterase. Prostaglandins of the E-series primarily increase the
levels of cyclic AMP via adenylcyclase stimulation (Tauber et al.,
1973). This increase in cyclic AMP by prostaglandins is not
blocked by adrenergic or cholinergic blockers (Strong and Bohr,
1967). Furthermore, bronchial smooth muscle contraction
induced by PGF_2 alpha does not appear to be mediated by SRS-A,
nor is it effected by 5-HT. This evidence further points to the
speculation that prostaglandins act on the lung cyclic AMP system
(Cuthbert, 1973).

Is there any interaction of prostaglandins and cyclic nucleotides? In general, it has been widely accepted that PGEs stimulate adenycyclase to increase cyclic AMP, whereas PGFs stimulate guanyl cyclase to increase levels of cyclic GMP. In view of the predominently opposing effects of PGEs and PGFs on many systems, this would be consistent with the concept of two opposing "forces," that is, cyclic AMP and cyclic GMP regulating cell function, which is the "yin/yang" hypothesis (Goldberg et al., 1975). However, these opposing pharmacologic actions of PGEs and PGFs have not been demonstrated in a variety of *in vitro* lung preparations. Stimulation of adenycylase-cyclic AMP system has always been obtained with PGE_1 and to a lesser extent with PGE_2, whereas PGF_2 alpha has significantly less (Tauber et al., 1973) or no effect. Prostaglandins of the E-series do not affect the guanylcyclase-cyclic GMP system, and the reported data on the action of PGF_2 alpha to alter this system are inconclusive. Cyclic AMP inhibits the immunologic release of mediators from whole lung or lung fragments, isolated mast cells, leukocytes, etc. A decrease in cyclic AMP, with or without an increase in cyclic GMP levels, enhances the liberation of mediators (Kaliner and Austen, 1974; Lichtenstein and DeBernardo, 1971; Tauber et al., 1973). The consequence of changes in the levels of cyclic nucleotides would be to alter the smooth muscle tone of airways and pulmonary vasculature as well as to modulate the release of mediators.

With respect to the calcium-mediated coupling of excitation and the contraction of smooth muscle, there is evidence that prostaglandins influence the release of bound calcium from cellular membranes (Higgins and Braunwald, 1972). Alteration of the membrane polarity might alter the contraction of smooth muscle. However, this theory awaits further elaboration.

CLINICAL SIGNIFICANCE OF PROSTAGLANDINS PERTAINING TO LUNGS

From the various experimental and clinical studies it appears that prostaglandins modulate both the respiratory and non-respiratory lung functions in health and disease. The hypothesis linking prostaglandins to histamine release and cyclic nucleotide actions on the cellular responses to inflammatory and immuno-logic agents is quite attractive (Kaliner and Austen, 1974; Tauber et al., 1973). Also, prostaglandins have been shown to possess a

bewildering spectrum of biologic activity in the lungs and other
tissues (Bergstrom et al., 1968; Hinman, 1972; Weeks, 1972;
Anderson and Ramwell, 1974) mimmicking inflammation and
immunologic reactions. Furthermore, diverse stimuli have been
found to release prostaglandins from lung, as previously pointed
out. Some of the pulmonary conditions where prostaglandins
have a role are discussed in the following.

Bronchial Asthma

The role of prostaglandins in bronchial asthma has not been
clearly established, although it has spurred the greatest interest
(Cutbert, 1973; Parker and Snider, 1973). Whether prostaglandins
are involved in the primary mediator release phenomenon of acute
hypersensitivity (Piper, 1973; Tauber et al., 1973) or is a secondary
phenomenon to the primary mediator release of histamine and slow-
reacting substance of anaphylaxis (Piper and Vane, 1971) needs
clarification.

Many pathophysiologic factors may be involved in asthma. The
tone of the airways could be viewed as an equilibrium between the
dilatory effects of epinephrine and PGE_2 and the constrictive
action of acetylcholine, PGF_2 alpha, histamine, slow-reacting
substance of anaphylaxis (SRS-A), other unidentified mediators,
and the α-adrenoreceptor effect of norepinephrine.

The role of aerosolized prostaglandins has been discussed. Of
significance is the evidence that asthmatic patients are more
sensitive to the bronchoconstrictor effect of PGF_2 alpha (8000
times) and the induced bronchoconstrictor lasts for a longer
duration (Mathé et al., 1973). Furthermore, asthmatics also show
a greater increase in sensitivity to histamine. Mathé et al. (1973)
feel that this is highly incriminating evidence for the central role
of the prostaglandins in the pathogenesis of asthma, and
reemphasize that endogenous and locally formed PGF_2 alpha may
be an important mediator of acute asthmatic attack. Elevated
levels of PGF_2 alpha in serum of ragweed allergic patients adds
some support to this hypothesis (Okazaki et al., 1974). However,
this hypothesis is challenged on the basis of its inability to assess
the sensitivity of the test because of nonspecific irritative properties
of aerosolized prostaglandins coupled with marked irritability of the
airways of an asthmatic patient, and the lack of demonstration of
the beneficial effect of aspirin in these patients (Parker and Snider,
1973).

The demonstrated inhibition of the release of slow-reacting substances of anaphylaxis (SRS-A) but not of prostaglandins by disodium cromoglycate from sensitized guinea pig lungs is evidence against the involvement of prostaglandins in asthma. Aspirin and related drugs have been known to inhibit prostaglandin bio-synthesis. If PGF_2 alpha is a mediator in asthma, then aspirin-like drugs should be of some therapeutic value. However, the majority of asthmatics do not respond to these drugs. Instead, there is a small population of asthmatics who are sensitive to aspirin and other prostaglandin synthetase inhibitors (Smith, 1971). It is thus intriguing to consider the alteration in relative rates of prostaglandin E and prostaglandin F_2 synthesis by such drugs, depending upon the aspirin-responsive and aspirin-hypersensitive patients.

Several investigators (Sweatman and Collier, 1968; Smith and Cuthbert, 1972; Cuthbert, 1973) have demonstrated the therapeutic efficacy of bronchodilator prostaglandins E_1 and E_2 in patients with bronchial asthma. Since prostaglandin E does not work via the β-adrenergic receptor (Tauber et al., 1973), it might be effective in treating the epinephrine-refractory asthmatic patients (Shaw and Moser, 1975).

Pulmonary Thromboembolism

Synthesis of prostaglandins E_1 and E_2 from arachidonic acid in platelets can be triggered in many pathologic reactions (Bergstrom et al., 1968). Prostaglandin E_2 can enhance platelet aggregation, and thereby thrombus formation. Pulmonary embolism is associated with the pulmonary release of prostaglandin E_2 and F_2 alpha (Lindsey and Wyllie, 1970). PGF_2 alpha is a vaso- and broncho-constrictor. PGE_1 inhibits platelet aggregation and is a vaso- and bronchodilator.

In experimental animals, air and particulate embolization is accompanied by bronchoconstriction (Clark et al., 1970), and release of prostaglandins, primarily PGF_2 alpha (Lindsey and Wyllie, 1970; Piper and Vane, 1971; Said, 1972). Acute emboliza-tion of the canine pulmonary artery with barium sulphate is associated with an increase in pulmonary artery pressure and pulmonary airway resistance response without affecting the pulmonary artery pressure. This suggests *de novo* synthesis of PGF_2 alpha in embolization (Nakano and McCloy, 1973). Although serotonin released locally from platelets in thrombotic pulmonary embolism has been suggested as a cause of broncho-

constriction (Moser and Stein, 1973), platelet production of
prostaglandin E and F has also been documented (Smith and
Willis, 1971), thus making it tempting to speculate on the role of
prostaglandin release after thrombus impaction in pulmonary
artery.

Other Diseases and Disease States

Prostaglandin levels are increased in shock. This occurs because
the prostaglandin dehydrogenase activity is considerably reduced in
endotoxic shock (Nakano and Prancan, 1973) and the mediators
in shock, histamine, and bradykinin stimulate the release of
prostaglandins and rabbit aorta contracting substance (Palmer
et al., 1970). Endotoxin-induced platelet aggregation has been
observed to result in pulmonary hypertension (Pennington et al.,
1973).

During anaphylaxis, many biologically active chemical mediators,
such as histamine, bradykinin, slow-reacting substance of anaphylaxis, and prostaglandins, are liberated from leukocytes, platelets,
and other blood cells (Piper and Vane, 1969, Lindsey and Myllie,
1970; Lichtenstein and De Bernardo, 1971; Tauber et al., 1973).
In the isolated, perfused lung, antigenic challenge can release
histamine, slow-reacting substance of anaphylaxis, and
prostaglandins (Piper and Vane, 1969), producing marked bronchoconstriction. In view of the simultaneous release of many other
substances, it is difficult to assess the extent and nature of the
contribution of prostaglandins during anaphylaxis.

The role of prostaglandins in inflammatory disorders of the lung,
chronic obstructive lung disease, sarcoidosis, neoplasm, etc., has not
been evaluated. However, it has been suggested that prostaglandin
release from lung, not necessarily triggered by pulmonary disease,
elicited pathophysiologic phenomena in other organs, for example,
cutaneous vasodilation in carcinoid syndrome and migraine
(Bakhle and Vane, 1974; Sandler, 1972).

Hyperinflated guinea pig lungs have been demonstrated to release
prostaglandin E (Berry et al., 1971). This has led to the hypothesis
that the systemic hypotension seen in patients who are on
continuous positive-pressure breathing may be due in part to
increased amounts of prostaglandin E reaching systemic circulation
(Higgins and Braunwald, 1972). Pretreatment of dogs with aspirin
has been shown to prevent the hypotension significantly (Said,
1972).

Ventilation-Perfusion Regulation (V/Q)

Because of the evidence that hyperinflation induces prostaglandin release (Berry et al., 1971), and that certain prostaglandins dilate the pulmonary vasculature, it has been suggested that prostaglandins may be responsible for maintaining the ventilation–perfusion (V/Q) ratio (Cuthbert, 1973).

In conclusion, it has been shown that the lung participates in the synthesis, release, and inactivation of prostaglandins. The catabolism is rapid, efficient, and selective, and is predominently via the enzyme 15-hydroxyl prostaglandin dehydrogenase. Prostaglandins have potent pharmacologic actions on the systemic circulation and the lung serves as a regulator of the prostaglandin levels in the blood. Should this mechanism become imbalanced, diseases and disease states will result.

SLOW-REACTING SUBSTANCE OF ANAPHYLAXIS (SRS-A)

SRS-A is an acidic substance of low molecular weight (approximately 400 daltons). It is probably not a true lipid, but forms a loose association with lipid, protein, and other molecules, such as lecithin (Orange et al., 1973). The exact structure of SRS-A is unknown. Its molecule contains both hydroxyl and carboxylic acid groups, and it is biologically active in extremely small doses (Orange, 1974). Arylsufatases destroy the activity of SRS-A (Orange et al., 1974; Wasserman et al., 1975). This has led to the suggestion that SRS-A is a sulphate ester and the presence of sulphur in the SRS-A molecule has since been confirmed (Orange et al., 1974; Dawson et al., 1975; Wasserman et al., 1975).

The release of SRS-A from guinea pig and human lung is accompanied by the release of prostaglandins E and F, and their metabolities (Mathé and Levine, 1973; Piper and Walker, 1973; Liebig et al., 1974), and is dependent upon antigen–antibody reactions (Parish, 1967; Orange et al., 1971). However, SRS-A and prostaglandins do not arise from a common precursor (Dawson and Tomlinson, 1974). The cellular location of the release is not known, although some investigators claim that mast cells release SRS-A. The conditions for the release of SRS-A are similar to those of histamine, being under the control of cyclic AMP and cyclic GMP and involving a presterase, anaerobic glycolysis, and calcium (Austen, 1974). However, whereas histamine is released

from preformed stores, SRS-A is not stored, and hence its production and release must be simultaneous (Brocklehurst, 1962).
Furthermore, unlike histamine, SRS-A causes a prolonged
contraction of isolated smooth muscle, especially after a long
contact time (Brocklehurst, 1970).

The release of SRS-A during anaphylaxis, in human chopped lung,
is inhibited by β-adrenergic drugs (Orange et al., 1971), methyl-
xanthines (Kaliner et al., 1973), prostaglandins E_1, E_2, F_2 alpha,
A_1 (Tauber et al., 1973), cholera toxin (Kaliner et al., 1973),
disodium cromoglycate (Sheard and Blair, 1970), calcium lack
(Orange et al., 1974), and colchicine and cytochalasin (Orange,
1974).

SRS-A formed either in human or guinea pig lung tissue has
similar actions. It contracts smooth muscle from trachea and
bronchioles (Berry and Collier, 1964). However, the concentration
of SRS-A required to cause bronchoconstriction of human
bronchioles is much smaller, probably signifying its importance in
humans when compared with other species (Brocklehurst, 1970).
SRS-A has a pressor effect when given intravenously, and probably
is a reflex effect of bronchoconstriction. At least in the guinea
pig, the pressor and bronchoconstrictor effects of SRS-A are
probably due to the release of prostaglandins and rabbit aorta
contracting substance (Piper and Vane, 1969), since they are
blocked by aspirin-like drugs (Berry and Collier, 1964).

RABBIT AORTA CONTRACTING SUBSTANCE (RCS)
AND RELEASING FACTOR (RCS-RF)

RCS is a lipid-like substance with a short (2-minute) biologic
half-life (Palmer et al., 1973). It is a nonprostaglandin product of
endoperoxide intermediates related to thromboxane A_2 (Hamberg
et al., 1975).

RCS is always released from lungs together with prostaglandins.
A variety of immunologic, mechanical, and chemical stimuli result
in the release of RCS from the lung. Release of RCS induced by
anaphylaxis has been demonstrated *in vitro* (Piper and Vane, 1969;
Palmer et al., 1973), and *in vivo* (Palmer et al., 1973) in the guinea
pig lung. However, no detectable RCS has been demonstrated
when passively sensitized human lung tissue is challenged with
antigen (Piper and Walker, 1973).

Bradykinin, SRS-A, histamine, RCS-RF (Piper and Vane, 1969); anaphylatoxin; dihomo-γ-linolenic, and arachidonic acids (Palmer et al., 1973); and slow-reacting substance C (Vargaftig and Dao Hai, 1971) release RCS and prostaglandins from guinea pig lung. RCS release has also been reported following mechanical agitation of chopped human lung tissue (Piper and Walker, 1973) and in isolated embolized guinea pig lungs (Palmer et al., 1973).

Irrespective of the nature of the stimulus for the release of RCS, aspirin-like drugs abolish the release of RCS from isolated, perfused, or chopped lungs (Piper and Vane, 1969; Palmer et al., 1973; Fjalland, 1974). Release of RCS is also inhibited by mepacrine, whereas that caused by arachidonic acid is not, thus suggesting that bradykinin might be activating phospholipase A (Vargaftig and Dao Hai, 1972).

RCS is a vasoconstrictor of both pulmonary and systemic arteries and veins of several species (Piper and Vane, 1969; Palmer et al., 1973), and is a bronchoconstrictor of human bronchial muscle *in vitro* (Piper and Walker, 1973). *In vivo* actions of RCS are not known. Since RCS is a product of endoperoxide intermediate (Hamberg et al., 1975), it is postulated that its *in vivo* actions may be similar to that of endoperoxide.

RCS-RF is a stable substance, which when infused into unsensitized lungs causes release of RCS and prostaglandins, but not histamine. Its release induced by anaphylaxis (Piper and Vane, 1969) is not inhibited by aspirin-like drugs, thus suggesting that it is not a product of prostaglandin synthetase (Palmer et al., 1973). It seems to act in the pulmonary circulation to release other mediators and does not seem to act on isolated smooth muscle. *In vivo* release of RCS-RF is not known.

ADENINE NUCLEOTIDE

The lungs inactivate ATP by deamination and dephosphorylation to adenosine and adenosine monophosphate. Pinocytic vesicles on the surface of the capillaries have been shown to have ATPase activity, and are possibly responsible for the degradation of ATP (Smith and Ryan, 1970).

Adenine nucleotides are vasodilators. They are released from the muscle after trauma and account for the hypotension. If indeed the lungs inactive adenine nucleotides, then metabolic degradation in the lung of these acidic compounds may suggest

the protective role of the lung in shock (Ryan and Smith, 1971).
However, the metabolic degradation of adenine nucleotides in the
lung has not been confirmed in the subsequent studies (Ryan et al.,
1972).

THROMBOXANES

These are a group of nonprostaglandin endoperoxides derived
from arachidonic acid in the platelets and lungs. Thromboxane A_2
is a major component of the rabbit aorta contracting substance
(RCS) and is a potent platelet aggregator. Thromboxane B_2 is an
inactive, stable compound (Hamberg et al., 1975).

STEROIDS AND THYROID HORMONES

Since the discovery that glucocorticoids accelerate the appearance
of osmophilic bodies in Type II alveolar cells (Wang et al., 1971),
considerable interest has developed in the relationship between
lungs and steroids. The lungs, like other tissues, have been shown
to take up hormones for their own use as well as to participate
in steroid metabolism. Human (Ballard and Ballard, 1974) and
animal (Giannopoulous et al., 1972; Toft and Chytil, 1973) lungs
contain cytoplasmic and nuclear receptors for steroids. Fetal
rabbit lung (Giannopoulous, 1974) has been shown to convert
cortisone to its more active analogue, cortisol, thereby permitting
its binding to the receptor. Furthermore, it has been shown that
fetal human lung cells in culture (Smith et al., 1973) and the
isolated, perfused lungs of rats and guinea pig (Nicholas and Kim,
1975) are capable of converting cortisone to cortisol.
    Since Type II alveolar cells are the likely origin for the production
of lung surfactant, glucocorticoids have been shown to hasten the
production of surfactant by fetal lungs (Torday et al., 1975).
This probably suggests the role of steroids in the prevention of
newborn respiratory distress syndrome. Furthermore, the physiologic role of glucocorticoids, at least in part, can depend on the
pulmonary conversion of cortisone to cortisol.
    Animal studies have also shown that testosterone is also
metabolized by the lung (Hartiala, 1974).
    Thyroid hormones, like glucocorticoids, also influence the
morphology of Type II alveolar cells and the surfactant production.
In adult rats it has been shown that thyroxine accelerates the

production of surfactant and thyroidectomy has the opposite effect (Redding et al., 1972).

COAGULATION AND FIBRINOLYSIS

The endothelial cells of the pulmonary artery contain a plasminogen activator capable of initiating fibrinolysis (Todd, 1964; Warren, 1963). The precise location of the plasminogen activator within endothelial cells and whether or not the lungs are a source of circulating plasminogen activator are not known.

Tissue factor antigen or thromboplastin is also present on the plasma membrane of the pulmonary endothelial cells (Zields et al., 1972), and it is an initiator of the extrinsic clotting system. *In vitro* studies have shown that thromboplastin degrades angiotensin I and II, bradykinin, and substance "P" (Simmons et al., 1974). This has not been confirmed in experiments using intact lungs.

SUMMARY AND CONCLUSIONS

Recent research provides sufficient evidence that the lungs are an active metabolic organ. However, the evidence is still largely based on animal experiments, and hence the full physiologic and clinical implications are difficult to assess.

Apart from its respiratory function, the pulmonary circulation exerts an important control over biologically active substances. Selective metabolism of these substances by the lungs probably has protective and physiologic importance. Substances possessing the function of circulating hormones pass through the pulmonary circulation unaltered, and/or are synthesized, whereas, those with local or systemic delitirous effects are either removed or metabolized, and thus their concentration in systemic circulation regulated.

Endothelial cells of the pulmonary vasculature bear most of the responsibility where pulmonary metabolic phenomena occur. These cells are the bearer of surface enzymes. In many cases the pulmonary enzymatic specificity has been characterized and the cellular, subcellular localizations of these processes determined.

Among the amines, serotonin (5-hydroxytryptamine) is completely removed and noradrenaline is only partially removed during their passage through the lungs. Adrenaline, isoprenaline, dopamine, and histamine pass freely through the pulmonary circulation. The

role of the lungs in the handling of acetylcholine has not been
established. Serotonin and noradrenaline are metabolized intracellularly after uptake from the plasma and histamine is discharged,
following the proper stimulus, from the intrapulmonary stores.

Similarly, impressive specificities exist for the peptide hormones.
The lungs play a dominant role in the catabolism of bradykinin—a
polypeptide with potent biological activity. Other peptides, such
as angiotensin II, oxytocin, vasopressin, eledoisin, and substance
"P," are unaffected during their passage through pulmonary circulation to function as circulating hormones. Although the lungs do
not inactivate angiotensin II, they do participate in the metabolism
of this hormone. They are the principal site of conversion of
angiotensin I to angiotensin II by the converting enzyme located
at the endothelial surface of the pulmonary vasculature. This
enzyme is not only important in angiotensin II synthesis, but is
also a kininase. Vasoactive lung polypeptides go through the
pulmonary vasculature unscathed. The chemical identity of
these peptides and their biologic activity are not certain at present,
although they have been shown to be the dilators of the smooth
muscles of systemic and pulmonary vessels. Similarly, the
physiologic implications of renally active lung substance (LS) are
uncertain at present, although it has been shown to promote
sodium and water retention.

The lungs play an important role in steroid metabolism, as well
as taking up hormones in their own use. This is best exemplified
by their role in the conversion of cortisone to its more active
analogue, cortisol, and the influence of both glucocorticoids and
thyroid hormones on the morphology of Type II alveolar cells
and surfactant production. In disease states, the lungs can be a
source of numerous polypeptide hormones. The hormone-secreting
potential of the lung is best exemplified by the ectopic endocrine
syndromes in a variety of pulmonary malignant and nonmalignant
disease states.

Acidic compounds, such as prostaglandins and nucleotides, pro-
vode another example of the selectivity of the pulmonary vascular
bed. The lungs not only participate in the synthesis and release of
prostaglandins, but also play a dominant role in their catabolism.
Unlike prostaglandin A, which escapes degradation during its
passage through the pulmonary circulation, prostaglandins E and F
are almost totally catabolized by the enzyme prostaglandin
dehydrogenase. Furthermore, the substrate specificity of the
enzyme is greater for prostaglandin E than for prostaglandin F.
By regulating the levels of prostaglandins E and F, the lungs

indirectly maintain the tone of smooth muscles of the airways and pulmonary vasculature as well as the ventilation–perfusion relationship. Prostaglandin A, by being unaffected during its passage through the pulmonary circulation, probably serves the role of a circulating hormone in the regulation of renal function. The lungs probably inactivate adenine nucleotides at the endothelial surface and thereby control the levels of this hypotensive substance.

The lungs also secrete vasoactive substances. These are not circulating hormones, but once released they could produce either local alterations in function, such as increased airway resistance, reduced lung compliance, and increased pulmonary artery pressure, or could result in systemic manifestations. A variety of immunologic, mechanical, and chemical stimuli and disease states may result in increased synthesis and release of abnormally large amounts of these hormones.

During anaphylaxis, many mediators are released into the circulation from their intrapulmonary stores (Piper, 1977). Though histamine is a major mediator of anaphylaxis, other mediators released are slow-reacting substance of anaphylaxis (SRS-A), prostaglandins E and F, eosinophil chemotactic factor of anaphylaxis (ECFA), kallikrein (which, upon activation, liberates bradykinin), rabbit aorta contracting substance (RCS), rabbit aorta contracting substance releasing factor (RCS-RF), serotonin, and others. Furthermore, components of anaphylactic release, such as bradykinin, histamine, SRS-A, anaphylatoxin, arachidonic acid, and dihomo-γ-linolensic acid, cause the release of prostaglandins and rabbit aorta contacting substance from the lungs. It is postulated that agents that influence the release of these mediators do so by altering the levels of intracellular cyclic AMP; a rise in concentration guards and a depletion of cyclic AMP promotes the release of these mediators.

Mechanical distension of isolated lungs, hyperinflation and hyperventilation *in vivo*, artificial pulmonary emboli, and pulmonary edema (Said, 1977) have been shown to be associated with prostaglandin release. In many cases prostaglandins are liberated along with other active mediators, such as rabbit aorta contracting substance, serotonin, and histamine in pulmonary embolism and vasoactive intestinal polypeptide in pulmonary edema.

Alveolar hypoxia has been known to result in pulmonary vasoconstriction. Prostaglandins, spasmogenic lung peptides (vasoactive lung polypeptide), histamine, and serotonin are considered to be the mediators released in alveolar hypoxia responsible for hypoxic pulmonary hypertension.

The lungs are a source of many polypeptide hormones, amines, and possibly prostaglandins in various malignant and nonmalignant diseases of the lung.

The lungs are also considered to be the source of potent platelet aggregator, the thromboxanes. They also possibly participate in coagulation and fibrinolysis.

ACKNOWLEDGMENT

The authors gratefully acknowledge the splendid assistance of Mrs. Elaine Riskin in typing this manuscript.

ABBREVIATIONS

ACTH	: Adrenocorticotrophic hormone
ADH	: Antiduiretic hormone (vasopressin)
AMP	: Adenosine monophosphate
cyclic AMP	: Cyclic 3′, 5′-adenosine monophosphate
APUD	: Amine precursor uptake decarboxylation
ATP	: Adenosine triphosphate
ATPase	: Adenosine triphosphatase
BAL	: 2:3 dimercapto propanol
BPF	: Bradykinin potentiating factor
Ca++	: Calcium
CRF	: Corticotropin releasing factor
DFP	: Di-isopropyl fluorophosphate
DG	: Deoxyglucose
D_2O	: Duetrium oxide
DPP	: Diphloretin phosphate
ECFA	: Eosinophil chemotactic factor of anaphylaxis
EDTA	: Ethylenediaminetetraacetate
FSH	: Follicle-stimulating hormone
Cyclic GMP	: Cyclic 3′, 5′-guanosine monophosphate
HCG	: Human chorionic gonadotropin
HGH	: Human growth hormone
HPL	: Human placental lactogen
5-HT	: 5-Hydroxytryptamine (serotonin)
IgE	: Immunoglobulin E
LH	: Luetinizing hormone
LS	: Lung substance

ME	: Mercaptoethanol
MSH	: Melanocyte-stimulating hormone
NE	: Norepinephrine (noradrenaline)
PG	: Prostaglandin
PGs	: Prostaglandins
PGE	: Prostaglandins of E-series (E_1, E_2)
PGF	: Prostaglandins of F-series (F_1, F_2)
PGF (alpha)	: Prostaglandins of F-series (alpha)
PG-dehydrogenase	: Prostaglandin dehydrogenase
PG-synthetase	: Prostaglandin synthetase
PTH	: Parathormone
RCS	: Rabbit aorta contracting substance
RCSRF	: Rabbit aorta contracting substance releasing factor
SRS-A	: Slow-reacting substance of anaphylaxis
V/Q	: Ventilation–perfusion
VIP	: Vasoactive intestinal polypeptide

REFERENCES

Alabaster, V.A. (1977). Inactivation of endogenous amines. Metabolic functions of the lung. *In* Y.S. Bakhle and J.R. Vane (Eds.), *Lung Biology in Health and Disease*, Vol. 4. New York, Basel: Marcel Dekker, Inc., p. 21.

Alabaster, V.A., and Bakhle, Y.S. Removal of 5-hydroxytryptamine in the pulmonary circulation of rat isolated lung. *Br. J. Pharmacol.* 1970; 40:468–482.

Alabaster, V.A., and Bakhle, Y.S. Converting enzyme and bradykinase in the lung. *Cir. Res.* 1972a; 31 (Suppl. II):72–81.

Alabaster, V.A., and Bakhle, Y.S. Inactivation of bradykinin in the pulmonary circulation of isolated lungs. *Br. J. Pharmacol.* 1972b; 45:299–309.

Alabaster, V.A., and Bakhle, Y.S. The bradykinase activities of the extracts of the dog lung. *Br. J. Pharmacol.* 1973a; 47:799–807.

Alabaster, V.A., and Bakhle, Y.S. Removal of nor-adrenaline in the pulmonary circulation of rat isolated lungs. *Br. J. Pharmacol.* 1973b; 47:325–331.

Anderson, N., and Ramwell, P. Biological aspects of prostaglandins. *Arch. Int. Med.* 1974; 133:30–50.

Anggard, E. Distribution of 15-hydroxyl prostaglandin dehydrogenase and prostaglandin Δ-13 reductase in tissues of the swine. *Acta Physiol. Scand.* 1971; 81:396–404.

Anggard, E., and Samuelsson, B. Biosynthesis of prostaglandins from arachidonic acid in guinea pig lung. *J. Biol. Chem.* 1965; 240:3518–3521.

Anggard, E., and Samuelsson, B. The metabolism of prostaglandins in lung tissue. *Proc. Nobel Symp.* 1967; 2:97–105.

Austen, K.F. (1974). A review of immunological, biochemical and pharmacological factors in the release of chemical mediators in the human lung. *In* K.F. Austen and M. Lichtenstein (Eds.), *Asthma, Physiology, Immunology, Pharmacology and Treatment.* London: Academic Press, pp. 109-122.

Ayvazian, L.F., Schneider, B., Gerwitz, G., and Yalow, R.S. Ectopic production of "big" ACTH in carcinoma of lung. Its clinical usefulness as a biologic marker. *Am. Rev. Resp. Dis.* 1975; 111:279-287.

Bakhle, Y.S. Inhibition of angiotensin I converting enzyme by venom peptides. *Br. J. Pharmacol.* 1971; 43:252-254.

Bakhle, Y.S., and Block, A.J. Effects of halothane on pulmonary inactivation of nor-adrenaline and PGE_2 in anaesthesised dogs. *Clin. Sci. Molec. Med.* 1976; 58:87-90.

Bakhle, Y.S., Reynard, A.M., and Vane, J.R. Metabolism of the angiotensins in isolated perfused tissues. *Nature* 1969; 222:956-959.

Bakhle, Y.S., and Vane, J.R. Pharmocokinetic function of pulmonary circulation. *Physiol. Rev.* 1974; 54:1007-1045.

Ballard, P.L., and Ballard, R.A. Cytoplasmic receptors for glucocorticoids in lung of human fetus and neonate. *J. Clin. Invest.* 1974; 53:477-486.

Barter, F.C. (1973). *The Syndrome of Inappropriate Antidiuretic Hormone.* D.M. (Nov.), Year Book Medical Publication, pp. 1-47.

Baumgartner, H.R., and Born, G.V.R. Effect of 5-hydroxtryptamine on platelet aggregation. *Nature* (London) 1968; 218:13-141.

Beck, C., and Burger, H.G. Evidence for the presence of immunoreactive growth hormone in cancers of lung and stomach. *Cancer* 1972; 30:75-79.

Bergstrom, S., Carlson, L.A., and Weeks, J.R. The prostaglandins. A family of biologically active lipids. *Pharmacol. Rev.* 1968; 20:1-48.

Berry, E.M., Edmonds, J.F., and Wyllie, J.H. Release of prostaglandin E_2 and unidentified factors from ventilated lungs. *Br. J. Surg.* 1971; 58:189-192.

Berry, P.A., and Collier, H.O.J. Bronchoconstrictor action and antagonism of slow reaching substance from anaphylaxis of guinea pig lung. *Br. J. Pharmacol.* 1964; 23:201-216.

Biron, P., Boileau, J.C., and Campeau, L. Norepinephrine inactivation in the pulmonary circulation of animals and human. *Clin. Res.* 1969; 17:230.

Biron, P., Campeau, L., and David, P. Fate of angiotensin I and II in the pulmonary circulation. *Am. J. Card.* 1969; 24:544-547.

Boileau, J.C., Campeau, L., and Biron, P. Pulmonary fate of histamine, isoproterenol, physalaemen and substance 'P'. *Can. J. Physiol. Pharmacol.* 1970; 48:681-684.

Boileau, J.C., Campeau, L., and Biron, P. Comparative pulmonary fate of intravenous epinephrine. *Rev. Can. Biol.* 1971; 30:281-286.

Boileau, J.C., Campeau. L., and Biron, P. Pulmonary fate of intravenous norepinephrine. *Rev. Can. Biol.* 1972; 31:185-192.

Boileau, J.C., Crevells, C., and Biron, P. Free pulmonary passage of dopamine. *Rev. Can. Biol.* 1972; 31:69-72.

Brocklehurst, W.E. Slow reacting substance of anaphylaxis and related substances. *Prog. Allergy* 1962; 6:539-558.

Brocklehurst, W.E. (1970). The role of slow reacting substance in asthma. *In* M.H. Harper and S.B. Simmonds (Eds.), *Advances in Drug Research,* Vol. 5. London, New York: Academic Press, pp. 109-113.

Brody, M.J., and Kadowitz, P.J. Prostaglandins as modulators of autonomic nervous system. *Fed. Proc.* 1974; 33:48-60.

Bryant, D.H. The syndrome of inappropriate secretion of antidiuretic hormone in infectious pulmonary disease. *Med. J. Aust.* 1972; 1:1285-1288.

Burack, B., Marcus, D., Miamoto, A., et al. Response of class IV patients to alpha blockade prior to open heart surgery. *Am. Heart J.* 1972; 84:456-462.

Caldwell, P.R., Seegal, B.C., Hsu, K.C., et al. Angiotensin converting enzyme. Vascular endothelial localization. *Science* 1976; 191:1050-1051.

Carlson, L.A., Ekelung, L., and Oro, L. Circulatory and respiratory effects of different doses of prostaglandin E_1 in man. *Acta Physiol. Scand.* 1969; 75:161-169.

Clark, S.W., Graf, P., and Nadel, J. *In vivo* visualization of small airway constriction after pulmonary microembolism in cats and dogs. *J. Appl. Physiol.* 1970; 29:646-650.

Collier, H.O.J. Endogenous bronchoactive substances and their antagonism. *Adv. Drug Res.* 1970; 5:95.

Collier, J.G., Robinson, B.F., and Vane, J.R. Reduction of pressor effects of angiotensin I in man by synthetic nonapeptide (SQ 20881 or BPP9a) which inhibits converting enzyme. *Lancet* 1973; 1:72-74.

Cotrell, J.C., Becker, K.L., Mathews, M.J., and Moore, C. The histology of gonadotropin secreting bronchogenic carcinoma. *Am. J. Clin. Pathol.* 1969; 52:720-725.

Crutchley, D.J., and Piper, P.J. Prostaglandin inactivation in guinea pig lung and its inhibition. *Br. J. Pharmacol.* 1974; 53:467 p.

Cushman, D.W., and Cheung, H.S. Spectrophotometric assay and properties of lung angiotensin-converting enzyme of rabbit lung. *Bioch. Pharmacol.* 1971; 20:1637-1648.

Cuthbert, M.F. Effect on airways resistance of prostaglandin E_1 given by aerosol to healthy and asthmatic volunteers. *Br. Med. J.* 1969; 4: 723-726.

Cuthbert, M.F. (1973). Prostaglandins and respiratory smooth muscle. *In* M.F. Cuthbert (Ed.), *The Prostaglandins: Pharmacological and Therapeutic Advances.* London: Heinemann, pp. 253-285.

Dailey, J.E., and Marcuse, P.M. Gonadotropin secreting giant-cell carcinoma of lung. *Cancer* 1969; 24:388-394.

Daughtry, D.W., Chesney, J.G., Spear, H.C., et al. Unexplained systemic manifestations of malignant lung tumors. *Dis. Chest* 1967; 52:632-639.

Davidson, C. Diabetes insipidus with an ACTH-secreting carcinoma of the bronchus. *Br. Med. J.* 1972; 1:287-289.

Davis, R.B. Discussion of the role of 5-hydroxyindoles in the carcinoid syndrome. *Adv. Pharmacol.* 1968; 6, pt. B:146-149.

Davis, R.B., and Wang, Y. Rapid pulmonary removal of 5-hydroxytryptamine in the intact dog. *Proc. Soc. Exp. Biol. Med.* 1965; 118:799-800.

Davis, T.R.A., and Goodfriend, T.L. Neutralization of airway effects of bradykinin by antibodies. *Am. J. Physiol.* 1969; 217:73-77.

Dawson, W., Lewis, R.L., and Tomlinson, R. The release of 35 S-labelled material and slow reacting substance of anaphylaxis from immunologically challenged guinea pig lung. *J. Physiol.* 1975; 247:37-38.

Dawson, W., and Tomlinson, R. Effect of cromoglycate and eicosatetrayonic acid on release of prostaglandins and slow reacting substance of anaphylaxis from immunologically challenged guinea pig lungs. *Br. J. Pharmacol.* 1974; 52:107-108.

Doser, F.E., Kahn, J.R., Lentz, K.E., et al. Purification and properties of angiotensin converting enzyme from dog lung. *Cir. Res.* 1972; 31: 356-366.

Dray, F., and Charbonnel, B. Radioimmunoassay of prostaglandin Fa in
    human plasma. Very low levels. *Prostaglandins* 1974; 5:173-174.
Eiseman, B., Bryant, L., and Waltuch, T. Metabolism of vasomotor agents
    by the isolated perfused lung. *J. Thor. Cardiovas. Surg.* 1964; 48:
    798-806.
Elliot, T.R. The action of adrenaline. *J. Physiol.* (London) 1905; 39:401-
    467.
Eltherington, L.G., Stoff, J., Hughes, T., and Melmon, K.L. Constriction of
    human umbilical arteries. Interaction between oxygen and bradykinin.
    Cir. Res. 1968; 22:747-752.
Engel, S.L., Schaeffer, T.R., Gold, B.I., and Rubin, B. Inhibition of pressor
    effects of angiotensin I and augmentation of depressor effects of
    bradykinin by synthetic peptides. *Proc. Soc. Exp. Biol. Med.* 1972;
    140:240-244.
Erdos, E., and Yang, H.Y.T. (1970). Kinases, bradykinin, kallidin and
    kallikrein. *In* E.G. Erdos (Ed.), *Handbook of Experimental
    Pharmacology.* New York: Springer, pp. 28-92.
Eyre, P., Lewis, A.J., and Wells, P.W. Acute systemic anaphylaxis in the calf.
    Br. J. Pharmacol. 1973; 47:504-516.
Fanburg, B.L. Prostaglandins and the lung. *Am. Rev. Resp. Dis.* 1973;
    108:482-489.
Favre, L., Vallotton, M.B., and Muller, A.F. Relationship between plasma
    concentrations of angiotensin I, angiotensin II and plasma renin
    activity during cardiopulmonary bypass in man. *Eur. J. Clin. Invest.*
    1974; 4:135-140.
Ferreira, S.H. A bradykinin potentiating factor (BPF) present in the venom
    of Bothrops Jaraca. *Br. J. Pharmacol.* 1965; 24:163-169.
Ferreira, S.H., and Bakhle, Y.S. (1977). Bradykinin and related polypeptides.
    In Metabolic Functions of Lung. *In* Y.S. Bakhle and J.R. Vane (Eds.),
    Lung Biology in Health and Disease, Vol. 4. New York, Basel: Marcel
    Dekker, Inc., p. 44.
Ferreira, S.H., and Vane, J.R. The disappearance of bradykinin and
    eledoisin in circulation and vascular beds of cat. *Br. J. Pharmacol.
    Chemother.* 1967a; 30:417-424.
Ferreira, S.H., and Vane, J.R. Prostaglandins: Their disappearance from and
    release into the circulation. *Nature* 1967b; 216:868-873.
Fishburne, J.I., Brenner, W.E., Braakasma, J.T., et al. Cardiovascular and
    respiratory responses to intravenous infusion of prostaglandin F_2a in
    the pregnant woman. *Am. J. Obstet. Gynec.* 1972; 114:765-772.
Fishman, A.P., and Pietra, G.G. Handling of bioactive materials by the lung
    (parts I and II). *N. Engl. J. Med.* 1974; 291:884-890, 953-959.
Fjalland, B. Inhibition by non-steroidal anti-inflammatory agents of the
    release or rabbit aorta contracting substance and prostaglandins from
    chopped guinea pig lungs. *J. Pharm. Pharmacol.* 1974; 26:448-451.
Flower, R.J. Drugs which inhibit prostaglandin biosynthesis. *Pharmacol. Rev.*
    1974; 26:33-67.
Freer, R.J., and Stewart, J.M. *In vivo* pulmonary metabolism of bradykinin,
    angiotensin I and 5-HT in rat. *Arch. Int. Pharmacodyn. Ther.* 1975;
    217:97-109.
Frick, M.H., and Virkula, L. 5-hydroxy indol-acetic acid excretion after
    pneumopnectomy. *Ann. Med. Exp. (Biol.) Fenn.* 1961; 39:101-103.
Fritz, A., and Overturf, M. Molecular weight of human angiotensin I. Lung
    converting enzyme. *J. Biol. Chem.* 1972; 247:581-584.
Gavras, H., Brunnet, H.R., Lavagh, J.H., et al. An angiotensin converting

enzyme inhibitor to identify and treat vasoconstrictor and volume factors in hypertensive patients. *N. Engl. J. Med.* 1974; 291:817-821.

Giannopoulous, G. Uptake and metabolism of cortisone and cortisol by the fetal rabbit lung *in vitro. Steroids* 1974; 23:845-853.

Giannopoulous, G., Mulay, S., and Solomon, S. Cortisol receptors in rabbit fetal lung. *Bioch. Biophys. Res. Commun.* 1972; 47:411-418.

Gillespie, E., and Lichtenstein, L.M. Histamine release from human leucocytes. Studies with deutrium oxide, colchicine and cytochalasin B. *J. Clin. Invest.* 1972; 51:2941-2947.

Gillis, C.N. Metabolism of vasoactive hormones by the lung. *Anaesthesiology* 1973; 39:626-632.

Gillis, C.N., Cronau, L.H., Greene, N.M., and Hammond, G.L. Removal of 5-hydroxytryptamine and nor-epinephrine from the pulmonary vascular space of man. Influence of cardio-pulmonary bypass and pulmonary arterial pressure on these processes. *Surgery* 1974; 76:608-616.

Gillis, C.N., Greene, N.M., Cronau, L.H., and Hammond, G.L. Pulmonary extraction of 5-hydroxytryptamine and nor-epinephrine before and after cardio-pulmonary bypass. *Circ. Res.* 1972; 30:666-674.

Ginn, R.W., and Vane, J.R. Disappearance of catecholamines from circulation. *Nature* 1968; 219:740-742.

Goffinet, J.A., and Murlow, P.J. Estimation of angiotensin clearance by an *in vivo* assay. *Clin. Res.* 1965; 11:408.

Goldberg, N.D., Haddox, M.K., Nicol, S.E., et al. (1975). Biological regulation through opposing influence of cyclic GMP and cyclic AMP. The yin yang hypothesis. *In* G.I. Drummond, P. Greengard and G.A. Robinson (Eds.), *Advances in Cyclic Nucleotide Research*, Vol. 5. New York: Raven Press, pp. 307-330.

Goldzimer, E.L., Konopka, R.G., and Moser, K.M. Reversal of perfusion defect in experimental canine lobar pneumococeal pneumonia. *J. Appl. Physiol.* 1974; 37:85-91.

Golub, M., Zia, P., Matsumo, M., and Horton, R. Metabolism of prostaglandin A, and E_1 in man. *J. Clin. Invest.* 1975; 56:1404-1410.

Granstrom, E. Metabolism of prostaglandin F_2a in guinea pig lung. *Eur. J. Bioch.* 1971; 20:451-458.

Greenberg, P.B., Martin, T.J., Beck, C., and Burger, H.G. Synthesis and release of growth hormone from lung carcinoma in cell culture. *Lancet* 1972; 1:350-352.

Gruby, L.A., Rowland, C., Varley, B.Q., and Wyllie, J.H. The fate of 5-hydroxtryptamine in the lungs. *Br. J. Surg.* 1971; 58:525-532.

Hamberg, M., and Samuelsson, B. On the metabolism of prostaglandins E_1 and E_2 in man. *J. Biol. Chem.* 1971; 246:6713-6721.

Hamberg, M., and Samuelsson, B. Detection and isolation of an endoperoxide intermediate in prostaglandin biosynthesis. *Proc. Nat. Acad. Sci.* (USA) 1973; 70:899-903.

Hamberg, M., Svensson, J., and Samuelsson, B. Thromboxanes: A new group of biologically active compounds derived from prostaglandin endoperoxides. *Proc. Nat. Acad. Sci.* (USA) 1975; 72:2994-2998.

Hartiala, J. Testosterone metabolism in rabbit lung *in vitro. Steroids Lipid Res.* 1974; 5:91-95.

Hass, F., and Bergofsky, E.H. Role of the mast cell in the pulmonary pressor response to hypoxia. *J. Clin. Invest.* 1972; 51:3154-3162.

Higgins, C., and Braunwald, E. The prostaglandins. *Am. J. Med.* 1972; 53:91-112.

Hinman, J.W. Prostaglandins. *Ann. Rev. Biochem.* 1972; 41:161-178.

192   *Chitkara and Khan*

Horai, T., Nishihara, H., Tateishi, R., Matswada, M., and Hattori, S. Oat cell carcinoma of the lung simultaneously producing ACTH and Serotonin. *J. Clin. End. Met.* 1973; 37:212-219.

Horton, E.W. Hypothesis on the physiological roles of prostaglandins. *Physiol. Rev.* 1969; 49:122-161.

Huggins, C.G., Corcoran, R.J., Gordon, J.S., Henry, H.W., and John, J.P. Kinetics of plasma and lung angiotensin I converting enzyme. *Cir. Res.* 1970; 27(suppl. 1):93-101.

Hughes, J., Gillis, C.N., and Bloom, F.E. The uptake and disposition of DL-norepinephrine in perfused rat lung. *J. Pharmacol. Exp. Therap.* 1969; 169:237-248.

Igic, R., Erdos, E.G., Yeh, H.S.J., Sorrels, K., and Nakajima, T. Angiotensin I converting enzyme of the lung. *Cir. Res.* 1972; 30, 31(suppl. 2): 51-61.

Iverson, L.L. (1967). *Uptake and Storage of Nor-adrenaline in Sympathetic Nerves.* London: Cambridge University Press, pp. 1-250.

Iwasawa, Y., and Gillis, C.N. Effect of steroids and other hormones on lung removal of nor-adrenaline. *Eur. J. Pharmacol.* 1973; 22:367-370.

Iwasawa, Y., Gillis, C.N., and Aghajanian, G. Hypothermic inhibition of 5-hydroxytryptamine and nor-adrenaline uptake by the lung. Cellular location of amines after uptake. *J. Pharmacol. Exp. Ther.* 1973; 186:489-507.

Iwasawa, Y., and Gillis, C.N. Pharmacological analysis of nor-epinephrine and 5-hydroxytryptamine removal from pulmonary circulation: Differentiation of uptake sites for each amine. *J. Pharmacol. Exp. Ther.* 1974; 188:386-393.

Jose, P. Niederhauser, U., Piper, P.J., Robinson, C., and Smith, A.P. Inactivation of prostaglandin F_2x in human pulmonary circulation. *Br. J. Clin. Pharmacol.* 1976; 3:342P-343P.

Junod, A.F. Uptake, metabolism and efflux of ^{14}C-5 hydroxytryptamine in isolated, perfused rat lung. *J. Pharmacol. Exp. Ther.* 1972; 183: 341-355.

Junod, A.F. The lung as a chemical filter. *Adv. Int. Med. Pediatr.* 1974; 36:1-18.

Junod, A.F. Metabolism, production and release of hormones and mediators in the lung. *Am. Rev. Resp. Dis.* 1975; 112:93-108.

Kadowitz, P.J., Joinei, P.D., and Hyman, A.F. Physiological and pharmacological roles of prostaglandins. *Ann. Rev. Pharmacol.* 1975; 15:285-303.

Kahlson, G., Rosengreen, E., and Thurnberg, R. Accelerated histamine formation in hypersensitivity reactions. *Lancet* 1966; 1:782-784.

Kaliner, M., and Austen, K.F. A sequence of biochemical events in the antigen incuded release of chemical mediators from sensitized human lung tissue. *J. Exp. Med.* 1973; 138:1077-1094.

Kaliner, M., and Austen, K.F. Cyclic nucleotides and modulation of effector systems of inflammation. *Biochem. Pharmacol.* 1974; 23:763-771.

Kaliner, M., Wasserman, S.I., and Austen, K.F. The immunological response of chemical mediators from human nasal polyps. *N. Engl. J. Med.* 1973; 289:277-281.

Kamakami, Y., Uchiyama, K., and Irie, T. Evaluation of aerosols of prostaglandin E_1 and E_2 as bronchodilators. *Eur. J. Clin. Pharmacol.* 1973; 6:127-132.

Karim, S.M.M., Sandler, M., and Williams, E.D. Distribution of prostaglandins in human tissues. *Br. J. Pharmacol.* 1967; 31:340–349.

Kay, A.B., Stechschulte, D.J., and Austen, K.F. An oesinophil chemotactic factor of anaphylaxis. *J. Exp. Med.* 1971; 103:602–619.

Kay, J.M., Waymire, J.C., and Grover, R.F. Lung mast cells hyperplasia and pulmonary histamine forming capacity in hypoxic rats. *Am. J. Physiol.* 1974; 226:178–184.

Knowles, J.H., and Smith, L.H. Extrapulmonary manifestations of bronchogenic carcinoma. *N. Engl. J. Med.* 1960; 262:505–510.

Konzett, H., and Bauer, G. (1966). The action of hypotensive polypeptides on the pulmonary arterial pressure. *In* E.G. Erdos, N. Back, F. Sicuteri, and A.F. Wilde (Eds.), *Hypotensive Polypeptides.* New York: Springer, pp. 375–384.

(Leading article). Pharmacology of the carcinoid syndrome. *Lancet* 1968; 1:404–405.

Ledingham, J.G., and Leary, W.P. (1974). Catabolism of angiotensin II. *In* I.H. Page and F.M. Bumpus (Eds.), *Angiotensin Handbook of Experimental Pharmacology.* New York, Heidelberg, Berlin: Springer-Verlag, pp. 111–125.

Lichtenstein, L.M. The immediate allergic response: *In vitro* separation of antigen activation, decay and histamine release. *J. Immunol.* 1971; 107:122–1130.

Lichtenstein, L.M., and DeBernardo, R. The immediate allergic response: *In vitro* action of cyclic AMP-active and other drugs on two stages of histamine release. *J. Immunol.* 1971; 107:1131–1136.

Liddle, G.W., Givens, J.R., Nicholson, W.E., and Island, D.P. The ectopic adrenocorticotropic hormone. *Can. Res.* 1965; 25:1057–1061.

Liebeg, R., Bernhauer, W., and Peskar, B.A. Release of prostaglandins, a prostaglandin metabolite, slow reacting substance and histamine from anaphylactic lungs, and its modifications by catacholamine. *Naunyn-Schmiedebergs Arch. Pharmacol.* 1974; 284:279–293.

Lilja, B., Lindell, S.E., and Solderen, T. Formation and destruction of ^{14}C-histamine in human lung *in vitro.* *J. Allergy* 1960; 31:492–496.

Lindsey, H.E., and Wyllie, J.H. Release of prostaglandins from embolized lung. *Br. J. Surg.* 1970; 57:738–741.

Lockett, M.F. The formation of a renally active polypeptide by cat lungs from alpha 2-globulin *in vitro* and the plasma concentrations of this peptide *in vivo.* *J. Physiol.* (London) 1972; 224:187–194.

Marrazzi, M.A., and Anderson, N.H. (1974). Prostaglandin dehydrogenase. *In* P. Ramwell (Ed.), *The Prostaglandins,* Vol. 2. New York: Plenum Press, pp. 99–155.

Mathé, A.A., Heolquist, P., and Hulmgren, A. Bronchial hypersensitivity to prostaglandin F_2a and histamine in patients with asthma. *Br. Med. J.* 1973; 1:103–106.

Mathé, A.A., and Levine, L. Release of prostaglandins and metabolites from guinea pig lungs; inhibition by catecholamines. *Prostaglandins* 1973; 4:877–890.

McGiff, J.C., Terrango, N.A., Strand, J.C., Lee, J.B., Lonigro, A.J., and Ng, K.K.F. Selective passage of prostaglandins across the lung. *Nature* 1967; 233:742–745.

Melmon, K.L., Cline, L.J., Hughes, T., and Nies, A.S. Kinins. Possible

mediators of neonatal circulatory change in man. *J. Clin. Invest.*
1968; 47:1279-1302.

Melmon, K.L., Sjoerdsma, A., and Mason, D.T. Distinctive clinical and
therapeutic aspects of the syndrome associated with bronchial carcinoid
tumors. *Am. J. Med.* 1965; 39:568-581.

Moir, D.C. Tricyclic antidepressants and cardiac disease. *Am. Heart J.*
1973; 86:841-842.

Moser, K.M., and Stein, M. (1973). *Pulmonary Thromboembolism.* Chicago:
Year Book Medical Publishers, p. 167.

Naito, H., and Gillis, C.N. Effect of halothane, nitrous oxide on removal
of nor-epinephrine from pulmonary circulation. *Anaesthesiology* 1973;
39:575-580.

Nakano, J., and McCloy, R.B. Effects of indomethacin on the pulmonary
vascular and airway resistance responses to pulmonary microemboliza-
tion. *Proc. Soc. Exp. Biol. Med.* 1973; 143:218-221.

Nakano, J., and Prancan, A.V. Metabolic degradation of prostaglandin E_1 in
the lung and kidney of rats in endotoxin shock. *Proc. Soc. Exp. Biol.
Med.* 1973; 144:506-508.

Needleman, P., Minkes, M.S., and Douglas, J.R., Jr. Stimulation of prostaglandin biosynthesis by adenine nucleotides. *Cir. Res.* 1974; 34:455-460.

Ng, K.K.F., and Vane, J.R. Conversion of angiotensin I to II. *Nature* 1967;
216:762-766.

Ng, K.K.F., and Vane, J.R. Some properties of angiotensin converting enzyme
in the lung *in vivo. Nature* 1970; 225:1142-1144.

Nicholas, T.E., and Kim, P.A. The metabolism of ^{3}H-cortisone and ^{3}H
cortisol by the isolated perfused rat and guinea pig lungs. *Steroids*
1975; 25:387-402.

Nicholas, T.E., Strum, J.M., Angelo, L.S., and Junod, A.F. Site and
mechanism of uptable of ^{3}H-l-norepinephrine by isolated rat perfused
lung. *Cir. Res.* 1974; 35:670-680.

Okazaki, T., Veriloet, D., Attallah, J., Lee, J., and Arbesman, C.E.
Prostaglandin synthesis and allergic reactions. *J. Allergy* 1974;
53:75 (abstract).

Omen, G.S. Ectopic polypeptide hormone production by tumors. *Ann.
Int. Med.* 1970; 72:136-138.

Omen, G.S. Ectopic hormone syndromes associated with tumors in childhood.
Pediatrics 1971; 47:613-622.

Ondetti, M.A., Williams, N.J., Sabo, E.F., Pluscec, J., Weaver, E.R., and Kocy,
O. Angiotensin converting enzyme inhibitors from the venom of
Borthrops Jararaca. Isolation, elucidation of structure and synthesis.
Biochemistry 1971; 10:4032-4039.

Oparil, S., Tregar, G.W., Koerner, R., Barnes, B.A., and Haber, E. Mechanism
of pulmonary conversion of angiotensin I to II in dog. *Cir. Res.* 1971;
29:682-690.

Orange, R.P. (1974). Formation and release of slow reacting substance of
anaphylaxis in human lung tissue. *In* L. Brent and J. Holborow (Eds.),
Progress in Immunology II, Vol. 4, Clinical Aspects I. New York:
American Elsevier, pp. 29-39.

Orange, R.P., Austen, K.G., and Austen, K.F. Immunological release of
histamine and slow reacting substance of anaphylaxis from human
lung. 1. Modulation of agents influencing cellular levels of cyclic
3′, 5′ adenosine monophosphate. *J. Exp. Med.* 1971; 134:136S.

Orange, R.P., Murphy, R.C., and Austen, K.F. Inactivation of slow reacting substance of anaphylaxis by arylsulfatases. *J. Immunol.* 1974; 113: 316–322.

Orange, R.P., Murphy, R.C., Karnovsky, M.L., and Austen, K.F. The physiochemical characteristics and purification of slow reacting substance of anaphylaxis. *J. Immunol.* 1973; 110:760–770.

Osborn, E.C., Tildesely, G., and Pickens, P.T. Pressor response to angiotensin I and II: Site of conversion of angiotensin I. *Clin. Sci.* 1972; 43: 839–849.

Overturf, M., Wyatt, S., Boaz, D., and Fitz, A. Angiotensin I hydrolase and bradykinase from human lung. *Life Sci.* 1975; 16:1669–1682.

Palmer, M., Piper, P.J., and Vane, J.R. Release of rabbit aorta contracting substance from chopped lung and its antagonism by anti-inflammatory drugs. *Br. J. Pharmacol.* 1970; 40:581p.

Palmer, M., Piper, P., and Vane, J.R. Release of rabbit aorta contracting substance and prostaglandins induced by chemical or mechanical stimulation of guinea pig lungs. *Br. J. Pharmacol.* 1973; 49:226–242.

Parish, W.E. Release of histamine and slow reacting substance with mast cell changes after challenge of human lung sensitized passively with reagin *in vitro*. *Nature* 1967; 215:738–739.

Parker, C.W., and Snider, D.E. Prostaglandins and asthma. *Ann. Int. Med.* 1973; 78:963–965.

Parkes, D.G., and Eling, T.E. Characterization of prostaglandin synthetase in guinea pig lung. Isolation of a new prostaglandin derivative from arachidonic acid. *Biochemistry* 1974; 13:2598–2604.

Pearse, A.G.E., and Polak, J.M. Neural crest origin of endocrine polypeptide (APUD) cells of the gastrointestinal tract and pancreas. *Gut* 1971; 12:783–788.

Pennington, D.H., Hyman, A.L., and Jaques, W.E. Pulmonary vascular response to endotoxin in intact dogs. *Surgery* 1973; 73:246–255.

Peskin, G.W., and Miller, L.D. The role of serotonin in dumping syndrome. *Arch. Surg.* 1962; 85:701–704.

Piper, P.J. (1973a). Distribution and metabolism. *In* M.F. Cuthbert (Ed.), *The Prostaglandins.* Philadelphia: J.B. Lippincott Co., p. 131.

Piper, P.J. Substances released from passively sensitized lung tissue during challenge. *Int. Arch. Allergy Appl. Immunol.* 1973b; 45:87–89.

Piper, P.J. (1977). Release induced by anaphylaxis. *In* Y.S. Bakhle and J.R. Vane (Eds.), *Metabolic Functions of Lung*, Vol. 4. New York and Basel: Marcel Dekker, Inc., pp. 261–295.

Piper, P.J., and Vane, J.R. Release of additional factors in anaphylaxis and its antagonism by anti-inflammatory drugs. *Nature* 1969; 223:29–35.

Piper, P.J., and Vane, J.R. Release of prostaglandins from lung and other tissues. *Ann. N.Y. Acad. Sci.* 1971; 180:363–383.

Piper, P.J., and Walker, J.L. Release of spasmogenic substances from human chopped lung tissue and its inhibition. *Br. J. Pharmacol.* 1973; 47:291–304.

Poole, S.W., Williams, E.D., Booth, C.C., Burke, C.W., Hartog, M., Anderson, D.C., Woodhouse, N.J., and Fletcher, C. A case of endocrine dysfunction with lung carcinoma. C.P.C. *Br. J. Med.* 1970; 1:281–286.

Puglisi, L., Berti, F., Bosiso, E., Longiane, D., and Nicosia, S. (1976). Ascorbic acid and prostaglandin F_2a antagonism on tracheal smooth muscle. *In* B. Samuelsson and R. Paoletti (Eds.), *Advances in*

Prostaglandin and Thromboxane Research. New York: Raven Press,
pp. 503-506.

Redding, R.A., Doublas, W.H.J., and Stein, M. Thyroid hormone influence
upon lung surfactant metabolism. *Science* 1972; 175:994-996.

Reilly, M.A., and Schayer, R.W. Studies on the histidine-histamine relationship *in vivo. Br. J. Pharmacol. Chemother.* 1968; 32:551-563.

Reiss, E. Hyperparathyroidism: Current perspectives. *Adv. Int. Med.* 1974;
19:287-301.

Robin, E.D. (1978). Humoral agents processed in the lung with extrapulmonary
effects. *In* E.D. Robin (Ed.), *Extrapulmonary Manifestations of
Pulmonary Disease,* Vol. 8. New York, Basel: Marcel Dekker, Inc.,
pp. 409-411.

Roof, B.S., Carpenter, B., Fink, D.J., and Gordon, G.S. Some thoughts on
the nature of ectopic parathormone. *Ann. J. Med.* 1971; 50:686-691.

Rosen, S.W., and Weintraub, B.D. Ectopic gonadotropin in bronchogenic
carcinoma. *JAMA* 1969; 210:908.

Rosenow, E.C., Segar, W.E., and Zehr, J.E. Inappropriate ADH secretion in
pneumonia. *Mayo Clin. Proc.* 1972; 47:169-174.

Ross, E.J. Hyponatremic syndromes associated with carcinoma of bronchus.
Quart. J. Med. 1963; 32:297-320.

Rubenstein, A.H., Zwi, S., and Miller, K. Insulin and the lung. *Diabetologia*
1968; 4:236-238.

Ryan, J.W., Neimeyer, R.S., and Goodwin, D.W. Metabolic fates of bradykinin angiotensin I, adenine nucleotides and PGE_1, and F_1a in
pulmonary circulation. *Adv. Exp. Med. Biol.* 1972; 21:259-265.

Ryan, J.W., Roblero, J., and Stewart, J.M. Inactivation of bradykinin in rat
lung. *Adv. Exp. Med. Biol.* 1970; 8:263-271.

Ryan, J.W., Ryan, U.S., Schultz, D.R., Day, A.R., and Dorer, F.E. Further
evidence on the subcellular sites of kinase II (angiotensin converting
enzyme). *Adv. Exp. Med. Biol.* 1976; 70:235-243.

Ryan, J.W., Ryan, U.S., Schultz, D.R., Whitaker, C., and Chung, A. Subcellular localization of pulmonary angiotensin-converting enzyme
(Kinase II). *Bioch. J.* 1975; 146:497-499.

Ryan, J.W., and Smith, U. Metabolism of adenosine 5′ monophosphate
during circulation through lungs. *Trans. Assoc. Am. Physiol.* 1971;
85:297-306.

Ryan, J.W., Smith, U., and Niemeyer, R.S. Angiotensin I: Metabolism by
plasma membrane of lung. *Science* 1972; 176:64-66.

Sachs, B.A., Becker, N., Bloomberg, N.A., and Grunwald, P.R. Case of
ectopic ACTH syndrome secondary to adenocarcinoma of lung. *J.
Clin. End. Metab.* 1970; 30:590-598.

Sadovongiwad, C. Pharmacological significance of biogenic amines in the
lung—5-hydroxytryptamine. *Br. J. Pharmacol.* 1970; 38:353-365.

Said, S.I. The lung as a metabolic organ. *N. Engl. J. Med.* 1969; 279:1330-
1334.

Said, S.I. The lung in relation to vasoactive hormones. *Fed. Proc.* 1972;
32:1972-1975.

Said, S.I. (1973). The lung in relation to hormones. *Basics of RD,* ATS Vol.
1, no. 3, pp. 1-4.

Said, S.I. Endocrine role of the lung in disease. *Am. J. Med.* 1974; 57:
453-465.

Said, S.I. (1977). Release induced by physical and chemical stimuli. *In* Y.S. Bakhle and J.R. Vane (Eds.), *Metabolic Functions of the Lung.* New York, Basel: Marcel Dekker, Inc., pp. 297-320.

Said, S.I., and Faloona, G.R. Elevated plasma and tissue levels of vasoactive intestinal polypeptide in the watery diarrhoea syndrome due to pancreatic, bronchogenic and other tumors. *N. Engl. J. Med.* 1975; 293:155-160.

Said, S.I., and Mutt, V. Polypeptide with broad biological activity: Isolation from small intestine. *Science* 1970; 169:1217-1218.

Said, S.I., Mutt, V., Yoshida, T., and Hara, N. Biologically active polypeptides from normal lungs. *Clin. Res.* 1975; 23:315A.

Said, S.I., and Yoshida, T. Release of prostaglandins and other humoral mediators during hypoxic breathing and pulmonary edema. *Chest* (suppl.) 1974; 66:12S-13S.

Said, S.I., Yoshida, T., Kitamura, S., and Vreim, C. Pulmonary alveolar hypoxia: Release of prostaglandins and other humoral mediators. *Science* 1974; 185:1181-1183.

Samuelsson, B., Granstrom, E., Green, K., and Hamberg, M. Metabolism of prostaglandins. *Ann. N.Y. Acad. Sci.* 1971; 180:138-161.

Sandler, G.E., West, D.W., and Huggins, C.G. Peptide inhibitors of pulmonary angiotensin I converting enzyme. *Biochem. Biophys. Acta* 1971; 242:662-667.

Sandler, M. Role of 5-hydroxyindoles in carcinoid syndrome. *Adv. Pharmacol.* 1968; 6, pt. B:127-142.

Sandler, M. Migraine, a pulmonary disease? *Lancet* 1972; I:618-619.

Sbar, S. Unilateral gynecomastia. *N. Engl. J. Med.* 1972; 286:1367-1368.

Schachter, M. Linins—A group of active peptides. *Ann. Rev. Pharmacol.* 1964; 4:281-292.

Schachter, M. Kallikreins and kinins. *Physiol. Rev.* 1969; 49:509-547.

Schayer, R.W. The metabolism of histamine in various species. *Br. J. Pharmacol. Chemother.* 1956; 11:472-473.

Scholz, W.H., and Biron, P. Non-identity between pulmonary bradykinase and converting enzyme activity. *Rev. Can. Biol.* 1969; 28:197-200.

Shaw, J.O., and Moser, K.M. The current status of prostaglandins and the lungs. *Chest* 1975; 68:75-80.

Sheard, P., and Blair, A.M.J.N. Disodium cromoglycate: Activity in three *in vitro* models of immediate hypersensitivity in lung. *Int. Arch. Allergy Appl. Immunol.* 1970; 38:217-224.

Silva, O.L., Becker, K.L., Primack, A., et al. Increased serum calcitonin levels in bronchogenic carcinoma. *Chest* 1976; 69:495-499.

Simmons, W.H., Burkholder, D.E., and Brecker, A.S. Effect of bovine lung thromboplastin on vasoactive peptides. *Fed. Proc.* 1974; 33:291 (abstract).

Skeggs, L.T., Kahn, J.R., and Shumway, N.P. Preparation and function of the hypertensive converting enzyme. *J. Exp. Med.* 1956; 103:295-299.

Smith, A.P. Response of aspirin—allergic patients to challenge by some analgesics in common use. *Br. Med. J.* 1971; 2:494-496.

Smith, A., and Curthbert, M.F. Antagonistic action of aerosols of prostaglandin E_2a and E_2 on bronchial tone in man. *Br. Med. J.* 1972; 3:212-213.

Smith, A.P., and Willis, A.L. Aspirin selectively inhibits prostaglandin production in human platelets. *Nature (New Biol.)* 1971; 231:235-237.

Smith, B.T., Torday, J.S., and Giraud, C.J.P. The growth promoting effect
of cortisol on human fetal lung cells. *Steroids* 1973; 22:515-524.

Smith, U., and Ryan, J.W. Pulmonary endothelial cell and the metabolism
of adenine nucleotides, kinins, and angiotensin I. *Adv. Exp. Med.
Biol.* 1970; 21:267-276.

Soffer, R., Reza, R., and Caldwell, P.R.B. Angiotensin converting enzyme
from rabbit pulmonary particles. *Proc. Nat. Acad. Sci.* 1974; 71:
1720-1724.

Spanos, A., and Spry, C.J. Inappropriate ADH secretion with chronic chest
infections. *Br. Med. J.* 1974; 3:785-786.

Starling, E.H., and Verney, E.B. The secretion of urinary 5-hydroxytryptamine
as studied on the isolated kidney. *Proc. Roy. Soc. Bi.* 1925; 97:
321-363.

Stewart, J.M. Role of lungs in the metabolism of circulating hormones.
Chest 1971; 59:7S-8S.

Stewart, J.M., and Freer, R.J. (1973). Inhibitors of pulmonary destruction
of bradykinin in the rat. *In* H. Peters (Ed.), *Peptides of the Biological
Fluids.* 20th Colloquim. Oxford, New York: Pergamon Press, pp.
331-333.

Steiner, H., Bahlback, O., and Waldenstrom, J. Ectopic growth hormone
production and osteoarthopathy in bronchogenic carcinoma. *Lancet*
1968; I:783-785.

Stjarne, L., Kayser, L., Mathé, A., and Burke, G. Specific and unspecific
removal of circulating nor-adrenaline in pulmonary and systemic
vascular beds in man. *Acta Physio. Scand.* 1975; 95:46-53.

Strong, C.J., and Bohr, D.F. Effects of prostaglandin E_1, E_2, A_1 and F_1
on isolated vascular smooth muscle. *Am. J. Physiol.* 1967; 213:
725-733.

Strum, J.M., and Junod, A.F. Radioautographic demonstration of 5-
hydroxytryptamine ^{3}H uptake by pulmonary endothelial cells.
J. Cell. Biol. 1972; 54:456-467.

Sweatman, W.J.F., and Collier, H.O.J. Effects of prostaglandins on human
bronchial smooth muscle. *Nature* 1968; 217:69.

Tauber, A.I., Kalmier, M., Stechschulte, D.J., and Austen, K.F. Immunologic
release of histamine and slow reacting substance of anaphylaxis from
human lung: V effects of prostaglandins. *J. Immunol.* 1973; III:27-32.

Taylor, D.M., and Siemsen, A.N. Bronchogenic carcinoma simulating hyperparathyroidism. *Arch. Int. Med.* 1965; 115:67-73.

Thomas, D.P., and Vane, J.R. 5-hydroxytryptamine in the circulation of the
dog. *Nature* (London) 1967; 216:335-338.

Todd, A.S. Some topographical observations on fibrinolysis. *J. Clin. Pathol.*
1964; 7:324-327.

Toft, D., and Chytil, F. Receptors for glucocorticoids in lung tissue.
Arch. Biochem. Biophys. 1973; 157:464-469.

Torday, J.S., Smith, B.T., and Giroud, C.J.P. The rabbit fetal lung as a
glucocorticoid target tissue. *Endocrinology* 1975; 96:1562-1567.

Turkington, R.W. Ectopic production of prolactin. *N. Engl. J. Med.* 1971;
285:1455-1458.

Turkington, R.W. The clinical endorinology of prolactin. *Adv. Int. Med.*
1972; 18:363-387.

Turner, M.A., and Horne, C.H.W. Primary fibrosarcoma of lung and diabetes
mellitus. *Br. J. Surg.* 1970; 57:713-715.

Unger, R.H., Lochner, J.V., and Eisentrant, A.M. Isolation of insulin and glucagon in a bronchogenic carcinoma metastases. *J. Clin. Endocrinol. Met.* 1964; 24:823-831.

Upton, G.V., and Amatrudda, T.T. Evidence for the presence of tumor peptides with CRF like activity in the ectopic ACTH syndrome. *N. Engl. J. Med.* 1971; 285:419-424.

Vane, J.R. The release and fate of vasoactive hormones in circulation. *Br. J. Pharmacol.* 1969; 35:209-242.

Vane, J.R. Inhibition of prostaglandin synthesis as mechanism of action for aspirin-like drugs. *Nature (New Biol.)* 1971; 231:232-235.

Van Euler, U. A depresser substance in fluid of the vesicular gland. *J. Physiol.* (London) 1934; 84:21.

Vargaftig, D.B., and Dao Hai, N. Release of vasoactive substances from guinea pig lungs by slow reacting substance-C and arachidonic acid. *Pharmacology* 1971; 6:99-108.

Vargaftig, B.B., and Dao Hai, N. Selective inhibition by mepacrine of the release of rabbit aorta contracting substance evoked by administration of bradykinin. *J. Pharm. Pharmacol.* 1972; 24:159-161.

Waaler, B.A. The effect of bradykinin in an isolated perfused dog lung preparation. *J. Physiol.* (London) 1961; 157:475-483.

Wang, N.S., Kotas, R.V., Avery, M.E., and Thurlbeck, W.M. Accelerated appearance of osmophilic bodies in fetal lung following steroid injection. *J. Appl. Physiol.* 1971; 30:362-365.

Warren, B.A. Fibrinolytic properties of vascular endothelium. *Br. J. Exp. Pathol.* 1963; 44:365-372.

Wasserman, S.I., Goetzl, E.J., and Austen, K.F. Performed eosinophil chemotactic factor of anaphylaxis. *J. Immunol.* 1974a; 112:351-378.

Wasserman, S.I., Goetzl, E.J., and Austen, K.F. Inactivation of SRS-A by human eosinophil arysulphatase. *J. Immunol.* 1975; 114:645-649.

Wasserman, S.I., Goetzl, E.J., Kaliner, M., and Austen, K.F. Modulation of immunological release of eosinophil chemotactic factor of anaphylaxis from human lung. *Immunology* 1974b; 26:677-684.

Weeks, J.R. Prostaglandins. *Ann. Rev. Pharmacol.* 1972; 12:317-336.

Weichert, R.F., III. The neural ectodermal origin of the peptide-secreting endocrine glands. *Ann. J. Med.* 1970; 49:232-241.

Williams, G.A. Elevated plasma calcitonin as a marker of bronchogenic carcinoma. *Chest* 1976; 69:451.

Winnacker, J.L., Becker, K.L., and Katz, S. Endocrine aspects of sarcoidosis. *N. Engl. J. Med.* 1968; 278:427-434.

Yang, H.Y.T., Erdos, E.G., and Levin, Y. Characterization of a dipeptide hydrolase (kininase II: angiotensin I). *J. Pharmacol. Exp. Ther.* 1971; 177:291-300.

Zields, S.M., Nemerson, Y., and Pitlick, F.A. Tissue factor (thromboplastin): Localization to plasma membrane by peroxidase-conjugated antibodies. *Science* 1972; 175:766-768.

Zusman, R.M., Snider, J.J., Cline, A., et al. Antihypertensive function of a renal cell carcinoma, evidence for a prostaglandin. A secreting tumor. *N. Engl. J. Med.* 1974; 290:843-845.

Index